2-16-07

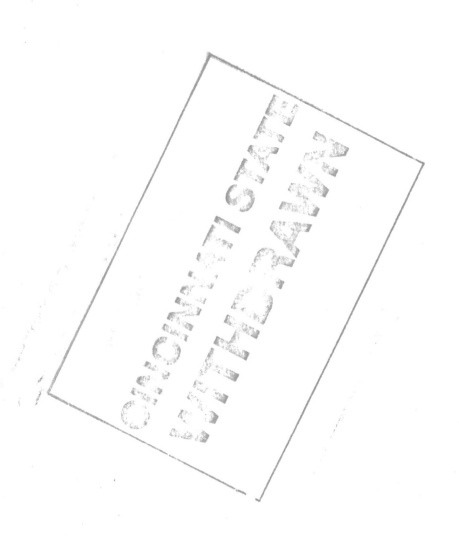

D1058728

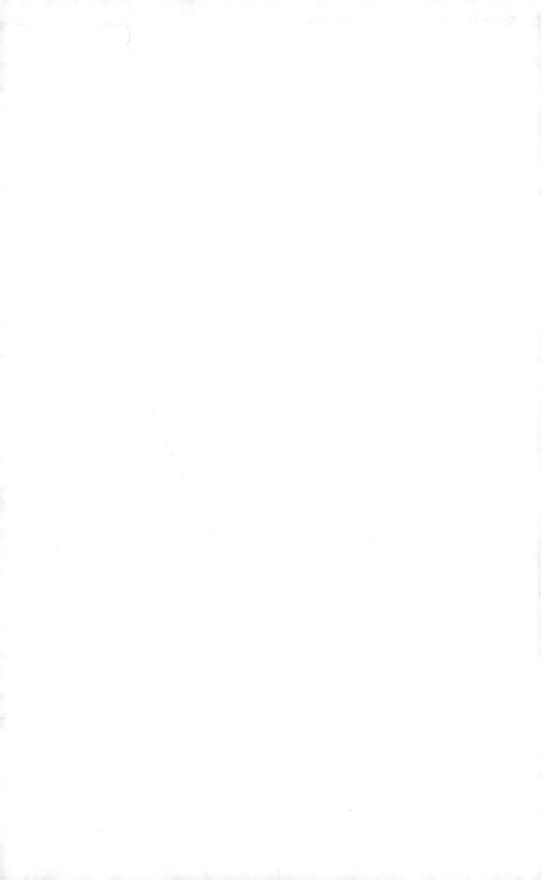

STEM CELLS

Recent Titles in
Health and Medical Issues Today

STEM CELLS

Evelyn B. Kelly

Health and Medical Issues Today

GREENWOOD PRESS
Westport, Connecticut • London

Library of Congress Cataloging-in-Publication Data

Kelly, Evelyn B.
 Stem cells / Evelyn B. Kelly.
  p. cm. — (Health and medical issues today ISSN 1558–7592)
  Includes bibliographical references and index.
  ISBN 0–313–33763–2 (alk. paper)
   1. Stem cells—Popular works. I. Title.
 QH588.S83K45 2007
 616'.02774—dc22   2006029481

British Library Cataloguing in Publication Data is available.

Library of Congress Catalog Card Number: 2006029481
ISBN: 0–313–33763–2
ISSN: 1558–7592

First published in 2007

Greenwood Press, 88 Post Road West, Westport, CT 06881
An imprint of Greenwood Publishing Group, Inc.
www.greenwood.com

Printed in the United States of America

The paper used in this book complies with the
Permanent Paper Standard issued by the National
Information Standards Organization (Z39.48–1984).

10 9 8 7 6 5 4 3 2 1

Contents

Section Three   References and Resources

SERIES FOREWORD

Every day, the public is bombarded with information on developments in medicine and health care. Whether it is on the latest techniques in treatments or research, or on concerns over public health threats, this information directly impacts the lives of people more than almost any other issue. Although there are many sources for understanding these topics—from Web sites and blogs to newspapers and magazines—students and ordinary citizens often need one resource that makes sense of the complex health and medical issues affecting their daily lives.

The *Health and Medical Issues Today* series provides just such a one-stop resource for obtaining a solid overview of the most controversial areas of health care today. Each volume addresses one topic and provides a balanced summary of what is known. These volumes provide an excellent first step for students and lay people interested in understanding how health care works in our society today.

Each volume is broken into several sections to provide readers and researchers with easy access to the information they need:

- Section I provides overview chapters on background information— including chapters on such areas as the historical, scientific, medical, social, and legal issues involved—that a citizen needs to intelligently understand the topic.
- Section II provides capsule examinations of the most heated contemporary issues and debates, and analyzes in a balanced manner the viewpoints held by various advocates in the debates.

- Section III provides a selection of reference material, including annotated primary source documents, a timeline of important events, and an annotated bibliography of useful print and electronic resources that serve as the best next step in learning about the topic at hand.

The *Health and Medical Issues Today* series strives to provide readers with all the information needed to begin making sense of some of the most important debates going on in the world today. The series will include volumes on such topics as stem-cell research, obesity, gene therapy, alternative medicine, organ transplantation, mental health, and more.

PREFACE

On a sultry Memorial Day in 1995, Christopher Reeve, an experienced horseman and rider, was catapulted from his horse to the ground during a jumping competition. Hitting headfirst, he fractured his neck and crushed his spinal cord exactly at the point it exits the skull. Reeve, known for his acting roles as Superman and in other films, became the inspiration for **stem cell** research and for hopes of regenerating damaged spinal cord tissue by implanting a unique group of cells that can grow new cells.

Why would Reeve promote a research idea that thus far has had no proven success? One word—hope—sums up everything. Stem cell research offers hope to millions who are victims of a multitude of diseases and disorders. In the United States alone, 16 million people, including hundreds of thousands of children, suffer from diabetes. There are more than 4.5 million people with Parkinson's disease, more than 5.5 million with Alzheimer's disease, and nearly 5 million with congestive heart failure. These numbers alone cannot describe the enormous suffering and personal tragedy of a child afflicted for life with type 1 diabetes who will eventually become blind and lose her limbs, of a mother who cannot recognize her children or grandchildren because of Alzheimer's, of a father imprisoned in a body wracked with Parkinson's disease. The people afflicted with these diseases are not the only victims. We cannot count the numbers of the relatives, friends, and health-care professionals who care for them daily who personally agonize at seeing their loved ones with such terrible conditions.

It is hoped that understanding the unique cells that can grow new cells will provide insight into the biology of life. The prospect that this may be a path to treating some of the most horrible human conditions provides motivation. Almost any disease is a target for stem cell therapy, but many questions remain. Is stem cell research an elusive target, and will it work? Is the means to the end—therapy and perhaps a cure for some people—ethical if other forms of life must be destroyed?

Stem cells have become the new darlings of the media. Stories about these mysterious cells are usually simplistic renditions of a complex subject. Although the idea of a "blank slate" that can form other cells has been theorized for centuries, stem cells hit the spotlight in 1998 when James Thomson published the first scientific paper on the topic in the journal *Science*. Since then, the field of stem cell biology has grown rapidly.

Although stem cells may hold the key to unlocking cures for scores of illnesses and diseases, they remain the most controversial field of scientific research today. Ethical questions as to the use and extent of embryonic stem cells and therapeutic cloning have divided people and spawned regulations on research.

This book is divided into three sections. Section One (Chapters 1–7) presents basic information that establishes the foundation for understanding the issues related to stem cells. Chapter 1 presents an overview—what stem cells are, why they are important, how they are classified, and descriptions of the types of cells. Chapters 2 and 3 trace historical events leading to current work in the field. Chapter 4 considers sources of stem cells and how they are cultivated in the laboratory. Chapters 5, 6, and 7 address procedures and experiments involving specific diseases and disorders that stem cell research may affect.

Section Two (Chapters 8–13) frames ethical and regulatory issues. Chapter 8 discusses the development of ethical precepts in history and notes how these principles relate to current problems in stem cell research. Chapter 9 discusses ethical considerations in the light of the twenty-first century, and Chapter 10 discusses religious considerations relating to stem cell research.

Chapter 11 of Section Two focuses on efforts at regulation by U.S. government agencies. Chapter 12 outlines the different perspectives and points of view of other countries and how their rules and regulations differ from those of the United States. Chapter 13 considers some future developments and ethical problems that may arise as progress is made toward understanding the processes of cell research.

Section Three concludes the discussion with a list of annotated primary sources, a timeline, a glossary, and sources for further reading and information.

This book on stem cell research is intended as a reference for students and lay readers. It attempts to describe medical and scientific concepts in common language. **Bold** type indicates the first use of key words, which are listed in the glossary at the end of the book.

Scientific Background of Stem Cells

Section One, consisting of Chapters 1 through 7, presents the foundations of the science that establishes stem cell research. This section of the book considers the historical development and scientific background of stem cell research, the growth and maintenance of embryonic stem cells, and the diseases and disorders targeted for research.

CHAPTER 1

Stem Cells 101

On Thursday, September 15, 2005, Mike Hagan, paraplegic since 2001, began to roll himself from Florida to California in a manually powered wheelchair to raise funds and awareness about stem cell research. Hagan lost use of the lower half of his body when a water taxi traveling at high speed slammed into his boat and broke his back in two places. He was transported by helicopter to Tampa General Hospital, where he saw paralyzed children struggling with the same problems he had. He admired greatly the efforts of Christopher Reeve to promote stem cell research, and when Reeve died in 2004, he knew he had to act. The Florida-to-California journey took him about 85 days; he divided the funds he raised between the Christopher Reeve Foundation and the Miami Project to Cure Paralysis.

Hagan trained for months and left his family for the grueling ordeal that took him through days of hot and cold to pursue the idea of stem cell research. Hagan's adventure is only one story that appears in the media about stem cells. Week after week, stem cells are in the news—more than singers, actors, and rock stars. But no one seems to know much about them. They are curious, mysterious, and unusual. What are these unknown blank slates that can provide the raw materials of life? Terms like *immortal, unlimited,* and *continuous* have been used to describe them. If these words are accurate, what does it mean? The goal of this chapter is to present scientific knowledge about stem cells, beginning with basic information about them.

WHAT IS A STEM CELL?

To precisely define the term **stem cell** has been a difficult task for researchers. A. G. Smith (2001) attempted this definition in an article in the *Annual Review of Cell Development Biology:* "Stem cells are defined functionally as cells that have the capacity to self-renew as well as the ability to generate differentiated cells." These cells have the amazing capacity to generate daughter cells that are identical to the mother cells, to renew themselves, and to produce offspring that can differentiate into other cells. This is the reason scientists refer to these cells as stem cells: many cells can stem from them.

Stem cells give rise to many different cell types that make up an organism. Thus, stem cells can develop into mature cells that have characteristic shapes and specialized functions, such as heart, skin, or nerve cells. They have the ability to divide or self-replicate for long periods; this replication may continue throughout the life of the organism. Stem cells can form many different types of cells that make up an organism. The ability to divide and form other cells is called **differentiation.** Another term that is used to describe this power to differentiate—this power even to change from one type of cell to another—is **plasticity.**

All animals (and even plants) have stem cells. In fact, most of what we know about stem cells has come from the study of mice and other laboratory animals. Understanding what makes stem cells "tick" has been the result of animal research. Although a human may receive a heart transplanted from a pig, humans cannot use the stem cells of other animals. The **DNA (deoxyribonucleic acid)** of each species is programmed to work differently. The possibility of repairing a severed human spinal cord or curing Parkinson's disease depends on the use of human stem cells.

Simply stated, stem cells are cells that have the ability to divide for indefinite periods in culture, and to give rise to specialized cells. The cells may be classified according to their origin as **embryonic stem cells (ESCs)**, **embryonic germ stem cells (EGSCs),** and **adult stem cells.**

As the name implies, embryonic stem cells come from **embryos** that have developed from eggs that have been fertilized **in vitro,** Latin for "in a dish or test tube" in a laboratory environment. These embryos, used with the consent of the donors, were leftovers from **in vitro fertilization (IVF)** clinics. Separated from the other parts of the early developing embryo, primitive cells can be grown in a culture medium to become embryonic stem cells. These cells are not derived from eggs fertilized within the body.

Embryonic germ cells are similar to embryonic stem cells except they are collected from the fetus later in development. The cells come from a region known as the **gonadal ridge,** which will later develop into the sex organs. Because the cells are farther along in the developmental process, they are slightly limited in their ability to give rise to organs of the body.

Adult stem cells originate in a mature organism and help maintain and repair the tissues in which they are found. These stem cells are responsible for replacing blood and tissues on a regular basis. For example, blood cells have only a 120-day lifespan; stem cells create new cells to replace the dying cells. One advantage in using adult stem cells is that small samples of tissues—or even the patient's own cells—can be used for implantation, avoiding problems of tissue rejection. Furthermore, adult cells do not carry the baggage of ethical issues that accompany embryonic research. Some scientists use the term **somatic stem cell** rather than adult stem cell.

WHY ARE STEM CELLS IMPORTANT?

Stem cells have three important characteristics that distinguish them from other cells:

1. They are unspecialized cells that renew themselves for long periods through cell division. They do not have any tissue-specific functions that allow them to perform specialized functions. For example, a single stem cell cannot beat with another heart cell; it cannot communicate with other cells, as nerves cells do.
2. Under certain conditions stem cells can be induced to become cells with special functions, such as cells of the heart muscle or insulin-producing cells of the pancreas. Unlike muscle, blood, or nerve cells, they can replicate themselves many times—a process called **proliferation.** A starting line of stem cells can proliferate in the laboratory for many months and yield millions of cells. If this happens over a long period of time, the process is called **self-renewal.**
3. Stem cells give rise to specialized cells. When this occurs, the process is called differentiation. Signals from both inside and outside the cell may trigger this differentiation. **Genes** control the internal signals. External signals include chemicals secreted by other cells, physical contact with other cells, and certain molecules called **growth factors.**

A future is envisioned in which stem cells may be used in treating diseases such as Parkinson's disease, diabetes, and heart disease. Such cell-based therapies form the basis of a new field—**regenerative or reparative medicine.** In addition, these therapies may be used for screening new drugs and understanding birth defects.

Stem Cell Backgrounder

To understand stem cells, one must consider that cells are the basic unit of living things. **Cell theory,** set forth in the 1850s, holds that cells are the building blocks of every tissue and organ in both plants and animals. With only a few exceptions, each animal cell has a nucleus, cytoplasm, and cell membrane.

The term **mitosis** is used to describe cell division. In this process, cells replicate exactly to make daughter cells that have a full complement of 46 chromosomes. The process of cell division proceeds as follows: Inside the nucleus are encoded instructions for the synthesis of **proteins,** in the form of a helical, double-stranded molecule called deoxyribonucleic acid (DNA). One might describe DNA as a genetic instruction manual made of many chapters. DNA makes a template, called **messenger ribonucleic acid (mRNA),** to produce molecules. The process of copying a DNA sequence to RNA is called **transcription.** A **transcriptional factor** initiates or regulates the process. Each kind of cell is structured to perform a highly specialized function. Bone, muscle, heart, nerve, and skin cells make up part of the organism, and each of these cells is distinct and different.

The **genome** is the organism's full complement of genes, or DNA. With the exception of the red blood cells and a few types of cells in the bone marrow, every cell has the entire genome. It is amazing that a cell in the skin has the complete genome of about 30,000 genes, as well as a cell in the muscle.

Meiosis is the process by which germ cells in the ovaries and testes divide to produce **gametes,** the generic term for sperm and egg. In meiosis the cells divide, and then divide again so that the sperm and egg have only half the original number, or 23 chromosomes. Meiosis occurs in phases. In phase one, chromosomes exchange genetic material so that they are not exact copies but may be mixed. In phase two, the cells contain two sets of chromosomes, which divide again to form half the number of chromosomes. These are packaged into sperm or eggs with only 23 chromosomes. At the point of fertilization, nature's arithmetic will come out right, with 23 chromosomes from the mother and 23 from the father making 46 chromosomes—the number required to form a human being.

Stem Cell Classification

Stem cells can also be classified according to their plasticity, or how versatile they may be in their development. The classifications may describe the cells' commitment to become particular kinds of cell: the **totipotent** stem cell, the **pluripotent** stem cell, or the **unipotent** cell.

Totipotent stem cells are the most versatile type. When sperm carrying the 23 chromosomes, chock-full of genetic material, fertilizes the female egg with its 23 chromosomes, the union occurs in the fallopian tube. The fertilized egg is called a **zygote.** This fertilized egg is said to be totipotent—from the Latin *totus,* meaning "entire." It has the potential to generate all the cells and tissues that will make up the embryo and support its development in the uterus. In mammals only the zygote and the cells resulting from the first few divisions have this all-encompassing ability to generate cells, the umbilical cord, and other structures. At this stage the cell is the ultimate mother stem cell, possessing potent **stemness**—the cell's potential to generate multiple mature cell types.

Pluripotent cells are like the totipotent cells in that they can give rise to all tissue types. Unlike totipotent cells, pluripotent cells cannot develop into an entire organism. On about the fourth day of development, the embryo forms into two layers that will become the tissues of the developing body. The outer layer will become the placenta, which in inner cells can form nearly any human tissue. However, because the cells cannot survive without the outer layer, they are now pluripotent, not totipotent.

However, Smith's definition of stem cells is not all-encompassing and applies only to embryonic cells. Certain adult progenitor cells and adult stem cells have reduced capacity for self-renewal. Unipotent stem cells are those cells in adult organisms that are capable of differentiating along only one line. The root word, *unus,* derives from the Latin term meaning "one." A limited number of undifferentiated stem cells are also found in the specialized tissue of the fully formed human body and are thought to function in the process of repairing. The definition of stem cells in general therefore must take into account the ability of cells to replicate.

The term *adult stem cell* is misleading because the cells can be found in humans of any age. Usually these adult stem cells are farther along in the process of differentiation than those found in embryos, meaning they can give rise to only a few types of cells in the body, not to all 200 types, as embryonic cells are capable of doing. Adult stem cells are most frequently obtained from human bone marrow, circulating blood, and umbilical cord blood.

HUMAN EMBRYONIC DEVELOPMENT

Three to five days after fertilization, the microscopic hollow sphere has about 50 cells and resembles a golf ball more than a human form. Still in the fallopian tube, it is now called a **blastocyst** (sometimes "blastomere") and is also totipotent, although this level of plasticity decreases rapidly.

The blastocyst from a five-day-old human embryo can give rise to only a limited range of cells. It is now pluripotent (a word derived from the Latin terms *plures,* meaning "many or several," and *potens,* meaning "powerful"). Still in the fallopian tube, it will now pass through several stages and form three layers—the **endoderm,** the **mesoderm,** and the **ectoderm.** This stage of development is called the **blastula,** when two kinds of cells—the **inner cell mass (ICM)** and the **trophoblast**—develop. Surrounding the cell is the **zona pellucida,** the outside cell membrane. The ICM will form the tissues of the embryo. The trophoblast will become the **placenta** and **chorionic membrane,** and will direct implantation into the mother's uterus. By the end of the first week, the blastocyst implants in the uterus (see Figure 1.1).

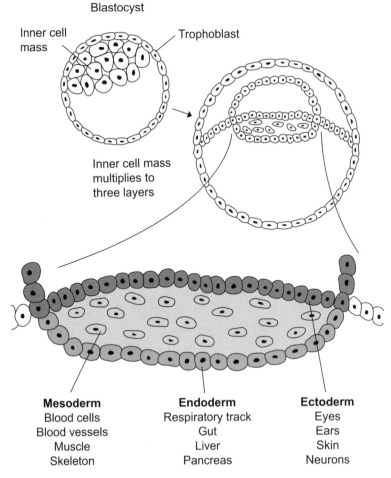

Blastocyst

Inner cell mass

Trophoblast

Inner cell mass multiplies to three layers

Mesoderm	**Endoderm**	**Ectoderm**
Blood cells	Respiratory track	Eyes
Blood vessels	Gut	Ears
Muscle	Liver	Skin
Skeleton	Pancreas	Neurons

Figure 1.1
Stem cell development. (Illustration by Jeff Dixon.)

Here an amazing feat of communication takes place. The cells begin to talk to each other in an intricate manner. They touch each other or in some way signal to tell cells to differentiate into certain other types of cells. Timing is critical in establishing the basic body plan for what shall become the head and what shall become the tail. This process is called embryonic **induction** and occurs in three stages: primary, secondary, and tertiary. Primary induction leads to the next stage, the **gastrula,** in which three germ layers are formed that become the differentiated tissues shown in Figure 1.1:

- Ectoderm—the outer layer that gives rise to the outer epithelium, including hair, nails, and skin; the sense organs; and the brain and spinal cord. Epithelium forms from the epidermis and other structures.
- Mesoderm—the middle layer that gives rise to bones, muscle, connective tissue, the circulatory system, and most of the excretory and reproductive systems.
- Endoderm—the inner layer that gives rise to the epithelial linings, those cells that form the linings of the body cavity, including the digestive tract, most of the respiratory tract, the urinary bladder, liver, pancreas, and some endocrine glands.

The process of the development of the three layers is called **gastrulation.**

Secondary induction involves a complex communication pattern to initiate the formation of the rudimentary brain and nervous system; tertiary induction regulates the development of body organs and other structures. The fertilized egg will continue dividing until it produces a complete organism capable of life in the uterus, or in utero. More than 200 kinds of cells will develop from a single, totipotent cell—the zygote or fertilized egg. These cells include neurons (nerve cells); **myocytes** (muscle cells); **epithelial** (skin) **cells;** blood cells such as **erythrocytes, monocytes,** and **lymphocytes; osteocytes** (bone cells); and **chondrocytes** (cartilage cells). Other cells essential for embryonic development include the extraembryonic tissues, placenta, and umbilical cord.

The blastocyst in vitro (i.e., in the laboratory) develops in a similar and predictable way. After fertilization, the embryo develops as follows:

- Day 1—Development begins 18 to 24 hours after fertilization.
- Day 2—The zygote undergoes its first cleavage to produce a two-cell embryo, 24 to 25 hours after fertilization.
- Day 3—An eight-cell mass called a **morula** that resembles a blackberry develops 72 hours after fertilization. Now the embryo begins to control its own development, and the mother's influences are reduced.
- Day 4—The embryo's cells hold close to each other in a process called compaction.

- Day 5—The cavity of the blastocyst is complete. The inner cell mass begins to separate from the outer cells, which become the trophectoderm that surrounds the blastocyst. This is the first sign of differentiation.
- **Implantation**—After about the fifth day, the human embryo makes a connection with the mother. This connection has been impossible to make in the laboratory, or even to monitor as it happens in the mother **in vivo.** However, scientists have studied implantation using the four processes of analysis of gene expression in small samples, in vitro fertilization, analysis of the clones of cultured embryos, and study of genetic markers. In humans, implantation occurs when the trophoblast cells invade the uterine tissue, forming a syncytiotrophoblast—something like a mega-cell. The fetus secretes proteolytic enzymes that dissolve the uterine epithelial cells and degrade the extracellular matrix. Implantation protects the embryo and provides its metabolic needs.

EMBRYONIC STEM CELLS (ESCs)

The embryonic stem cell is defined by its origin in the embryo. The fertilized egg has unbounded stemness. At this stage it is totipotent and can create all kinds of cells. Totipotency is limited to only one or two divisions. As the egg becomes a blastocyst and before it implants in the uterus, the hollow round ball develops a clump of cells—the inner cell mass—and becomes pluripotent.

Embryonic stem cells are harvested exclusively from this inner cell mass in the blastocyst. When placed in a cell culture in vitro, ESCs differentiate into many kinds of cells, which are shown in all three germ layers. But because the induction or communication process is disrupted between the ICM and the trophoblast, the cells can generate only embryonic germ cells that will not become a human embryo.

This remarkable feat of the ESC was first shown in the 1980s, using the ICM of a mouse blastocyst. In the culture dish, cell-to-cell communication led to the formation of nerve, skin, and other cells. But without the surrounding layers of the trophoblast, they received no signals from the mother's uterus. The cells became like wandering boys, able to make all the necessary differentiated cells but unable to put them together to become living beings.

ADULT STEM CELLS

The embryo usually becomes a fetus about eight weeks after fertilization. At this time another type of cell—the adult stem cell—emerges. The discovery that these cells were present in many formed adult tissues and organs changed the paradigm of past assumptions of how the body repairs itself. In the past, it was assumed that skin cells near the area of a cut or scraped knee would rush to repair the offended area. Brain cells, muscles, and some other cells were thought to never repair themselves. But recent research on adult stem cells has changed the picture. Adult tissues and organs have stem cells that are believed to play a role in the regeneration of damaged tissues and organs (see Table 1.1, Stem Cells in Adult Organs and Tissues). Chapters 5, 6, and 7 explore stem cell development and stem cell harvesting in each of the areas noted in Table 1.1.

The adult stem cell is undifferentiated and unspecialized. However, Table 1.1 shows that these adult cells do exist in specialized and differentiated tissues and organs. They can renew themselves and differentiate to

Table 1.1   Stem Cells in Adult Organs and Tissues

Body Part	Stem Cells
Brain	Stem cells here can become **astrocytes, oligodendrocytes,** and **neurons.** Some scientists theorize they may form certain blood cells.
Eye	Stem cells have been isolated in the cornea and retina.
Teeth	Stem cells have been found in the dental pulp of the teeth.
Bone marrow	These cells give rise to blood cells and the cells that become bone and cartilage. Blood cell precursors are called **hematopoietic** stem cells, and bone and cartilage cells are called **stroma cells.**
Skin	The largest organ in the body has stem cells that are related to the epidermis, epithelium, and hair follicles, which appear to be associated with repair and replacement.
Endothelium	Cells in the lining of the organs differentiate into blood vessels—arteries, veins, capillaries—and into the muscle of the heart. They are called **hemangioblasts** and may arise in the bone marrow.
Skeletal system	Bone marrow appears to be a promising place from which to harvest stem cells. These cells may be used during bouts of exercise or during the repair of injury.
Digestive system	Stem cells are known to repair problems and dysfunction in the lining of the intestine.
Pancreas	Although not yet proven, stem cells are believed to exist in the pancreas.
Liver	Although not yet proven, stem cells are believed to work to repair damage to the liver.

Source: Developed by Evelyn B. Kelly.

yield all the specialized cell types of the tissue from which they originate. For example, adult stem cells from the skin can form cells related to the skin, although they cannot form all the cells of the body like the embryonic stem cells can.

Embryonic stem cells are identified in the ICM, but finding adult stem cells is much more difficult. For example, in certain organs, they may be present in no more than one out of 15,000 cells. Although the exact source of these adult stem cells is unclear, three ideas have been proposed to explain their origin:

1. They are embryonic cells that were set aside when the tissue first developed.
2. They may be part of a migrating group of embryonic cells that became part of the organs or tissues during early divisions.
3. They may have developed after embryonic formation in some process of **dedifferentiation.**

The adult stem cells appear to be less plastic than the embryonic stem cell (ESC). For example, when both adult and embryonic stem cells were injected into mice, adult stem cells went to the area where they belong. Stem cells from the bone marrow gravitated there; those that were brain cells went to the brain. The ESCs did not go to any differentiated tissue but clumped together to form tumor-like masses. In addition, in the test tube, adult stem cells differentiate into only a small number of cells, while ESCs become many cell types representing all germ layers. However, several scientists are now challenging the dogma of the limited plasticity of adult stem cells.

While adult cells may lead to the first important therapeutic uses, embryonic cells present the possibility of devising therapies for most diseases and disorders. Testifying before the U.S. Senate Subcommittee on Stem Cell Research in 1998, Dr. James Thomson outlined a future made possible by embryo stem cell technology. He described how the cells could enable standardized production of large purified populations of normal human cells to provide limitless sources of tissue for pharmacologic research and transplantation therapies. Future clinical targets for the repair of blood, bone, and other tissues include blood cell repopulation, osteoarthritis, Parkinson's disease, diabetes, spinal cord injury, stroke, burns, and myocardial infarction. Study of embryo lines could provide insight into abnormal development that cannot be accessed in the intact embryo. These studies are having an important impact in clinical research on birth defects, infertility, and pregnancy loss.

Research using embryonic stem cells is controversial because it requires the embryo to be destroyed, invoking ethical questions for those

Table 1.2   Patients and Possibilities

Condition	Number of Persons Afflicted
Heart disease	58 million
Autoimmune diseases	30 million
Diabetes	16 million
Osteoporosis	10 million
Cancers	8.2 million
Alzheimer's disease	5.5 million
Parkinson's disease	4.5 million
Burns	0.3 million
Spinal cord injuries	0.25 million
Birth defects	0.15 million

Sources: Developed by Evelyn B. Kelly, based on Web sites of the U.S. Centers for Disease Control and Prevention, http://www.cdc.gov/ and various organizations.

wishing to uphold the sanctity of life. Adult stem cells are very important because they do not give rise to the ethical questions related to destruction of the embryo. However, the difficulty of harvesting them and their limited plasticity are major hurdles for researchers. The potential for U.S. patient populations to benefit from stem cell–based therapies is overwhelming, as shown in Table 1.2, Patients and Possibilities. Researchers around the world are working on the problems; when these are overcome, we may see the anticipated miracle cures.

Although research on stem cells seems to have developed only in recent decades, the idea of the blank slate of cells with the potential to take shape as many different types of cells has roots in historical thought. Chapter 2 traces the exciting ideas of how the slates of life were perceived in earlier times.

History of Stem Cells and Stem Cell Research Through the 1980s

In 1996 bicyclist Lance Armstrong was diagnosed with a rare kind of testicular cancer, known as a **teratoma** (literally, "monstrous tumor"). Because the tumor was caught in time, administering the chemotherapy drug cisplastin restored him to health. What does Lance Armstrong's cancer have to do with stem cell research? Locating and understanding the unique nature of teratomas was one of the important milestones in the development of stem cell research.

Three major historical trends established the current knowledge of stem cells:

- First were studies of reproduction, or how species reproduce. Locating the organs and processes of reproduction or generation gave researchers the impetus to speculate about the causes for development.
- Second were regeneration studies. Understanding how and why certain animals regrow damaged or injured parts generated questions about the origin of this unique feature intrinsic to some animals and not to others.
- Third, the nineteenth century produced a new science called **teratogeny,** or study of the creation of monsters. Results of teratogenic experiments led to speculation about stem cells.

These trends merged in the latter part of the twentieth century to create an explosion of stem cell research.

REPRODUCTION AND THE STUDY OF EMBRYOLOGY

Ancient writings of the Hindus and Greeks addressed the question of generation. The Manava-Dharma-Sastra, sacred code of the Hindus written between the thirteenth and fourteenth centuries BC, held that the fetus results from the mixing of two seeds from the parents. Greek philosophers believed that organisms could arise sexually, asexually (without sperm and egg), or by spontaneous generation (development that had no obvious cause). As early as the sixth century BC, Greek physicians suggested studying the embryo developing within the chicken egg to investigate embryology. Anaxagoras of Clazomenae and Empedocles of Acragas were fifth-century BC adherents of the Pythagorean school. Like the Hindus, they believed that the developing offspring was the result of the mixing of two seeds from the parents. According to Hippocrates (460–370 BC), the father of medicine, all parts of the body contain both male and female principles. Aristotle (384–322 BC) proposed two important models of development—**preformation** and **epigenesis.** According to the theory of preformation, a miniature individual is present in the mother's egg or father's semen and begins to grow when properly stimulated. Aristotle preferred the theory of epigenesis, which proposes that the embryo begins as an undifferentiated mass and that new parts are added during development. He believed the female contributed the unorganized mass through the menstrual flow, and that the male parent provided the form or soul, which guided development to form the first organ, the heart. This idea of the undifferentiated mass constitutes a rudimentary concept of stem cells.

Another school of Greek medicine was developing at the prestigious medical school at Alexandria. Herophilus (340–300 BC) proposed that women have testes and that the female genitalia are inverted versions of the male's. Fellow Alexandrian Soranus, a Greek physician of the second century, studied diseases of women and determined that females are imperfect versions of males. He believed that both sexes' organs are exactly alike except that the female's are inverted and inferior. The Alexandrians considered the female vagina to be an inverted, immature penis. Being inferior, the womb was considered an unstable organ linked to hysteria—from the Greek word *hyster,* or "womb." Crying, milk production, and menstruation supposedly showed that women were leaky vessels full of holes. Galen (130–210 AD), who emphasized the medicine of Hippocrates, determined that the seeds of both man and woman contribute to their offspring but that each one contributes only one principle. Galen also adopted the Alexandrian school's ideas of the anatomy of the female.

Glimmers of Change: The Renaissance

Throughout the centuries known as the Middle, or Dark, Ages, little was added to the knowledge of medicine. In the sixteenth century, even Andreas Vesalius (1514–1562), father of modern anatomy, echoed the idea that the woman's reproductive tracts were inverted versions of the man's organs and that the uterine tubes and seminal ducts were parallel. But Gabriele Fallopio (1523–1566), a student of the master anatomist Vesalius, was puzzled when he looked at the anatomy of female mammals. Vesalius had used only dogs to study the reproductive system, but Fallopio dissected not only male adult human cadavers but also those of women, newborns, infants, and children. He questioned the prevailing beliefs about women's anatomy that were based on the writings of Aristotle, Galen, Soranus, and the Bible. He saw tubes that were shaped like small trumpets, an odd-shaped structure that held a watery fluid, and others that held a yellowish fluid. Fallopio was the first to look at the fallopian tubes, which bear his name, and at the ovaries with their eggs encased in the follicle. Investigating reproduction was not acceptable at this time, but Fallopio laid the foundation for others to follow.

Curious Renaissance investigators contributed to the knowledge of reproduction. Known as the discoverer of blood circulation, William Harvey (1578–1657) also studied embryology and had doubts about many of Aristotle's theories. His teacher Girolamo Fabrici (1516–1619), who may be considered the father of **embryology,** inspired him to prove that epigenesis was a valid theory. Using deer that had mated, Harvey found no evidence of a developing embryo in the uterus until six or seven weeks after conception. He was convinced that generation must begin somewhere else. Many of Harvey's followers rejected epigenesis, and turned to the idea of preformation. Fallopio and Harvey were contemporaries, but it would be another century before the discovery of the process by which eggs are released from the ovaries to pass through the fallopian tubes to implant in the uterus.

Dutch anatomist Regnier de Graaf (1641–1673) began observing the structures of many animals, including humans. He is credited with naming the ovaries and finding the corpus luteum (yellow body), a structure within the ovary that secretes the hormone progesterone. The follicle around the egg is called the graafian follicle. However, he mistakenly thought the follicle was the egg.

For most investigators, studying the reproductive system was not a priority. As the seventeenth century unfolded, bitter disputes arose surrounding the philosophical and intellectual problems of generation. In Delft, the Netherlands, Anton van Leeuwenhoek (1632–1723) invented the microscope and went on to see in semen little animalcules or spermatic worms; he also observed the eggs of many species. Leeuwenhoek's discovery gave rise to debate among the ovists, who believed that humans were generated from eggs, and the animalculists, who believed that preformed individuals must exist in the sperm. The discovery of the microscope appeared to support the idea of preformation, an idea that held on for a century.

One eighteenth-century naturalist disagreed with the idea of a being preformed in either the egg or the sperm. Outspoken Casper Friedrich Wolff (1733–1794) published an article in 1759 titled "Theory of Generation" in which he argued that organs of the body do not exist in some preexistent form at the beginning of gestation but evolve from some undifferentiated material through a series of steps. Here was a better developed rudimentary idea for stem cells.

The eighteenth-century natural philosophy movement adopted many of Wolff's ideas, and led to the development of cell theory during the nineteenth century. Using careful observation and illustrations, Karl Ernst von Baer (1792–1876) studied egg formation in both humans and animals and was the first to note a resemblance between dog and bird embryos as they developed. Later in the nineteenth century, Belgian zoologist Edouard Van Beneden (1845–1910) described in detail the early phases found by Baer. He found that substances in the nucleus—later called chromatin—were reduced or divided during production of the gamete (i.e., the egg or sperm) in the nematode worm. Studying mammals such as bats and rabbits, he demonstrated how the zygote divided, or cleaved, to form a "blastodermic vesicle," now known as the blastocyst. He also described the three basic germ layers.

Toward the end of the nineteenth century Wilhelm Roux (1850–1924) founded a new discipline—developmental mechanics—that argued for embryologists to adapt experimental tools and the laws of chemistry and physics to analyze development. Roux questioned whether the embryo developed through self-differentiation or correlative-dependent differentiation. Self-differentiation is the capacity of the egg or any part of the embryo to develop independently of the parts around it; correlative-dependent differentiation means development is dependent on extraneous stimuli in other parts of the embryo. Roux performed a famous experiment in which he destroyed one of the cells of a frog embryo at the two-cell stage. The damaged cell developed into a half–embryo, thus supporting

Roux's belief that each cell develops independently of its neighboring cells. However, others who repeated Roux's experiments came to different conclusions. Hans Adolph Dreisch (1869–1941), experimenting with eggs of the sea urchin, concluded that at some level all parts of the embryo were uniform and that the result of any given cell was a function of the whole.

Albert Brachet (1869–1930), a colleague of Van Beneden, founded the famous Brussels school of embryology that supported strongly the ideas of the new science of developmental mechanics and added the idea of phylogenetic, or causal, embryology. Brachet was the first to keep a rabbit blastocyst alive and developing outside the body for 48 hours in blood plasma.

Inspired by the ideas of Charles Darwin, the Brussels school that was speculating on many mammals' early development proposed the idea that ontogeny recapitulates phylogeny. This concept theorizes that the development of the embryo follows the development of the evolution of the species. Interest in phylogenetic embryology continued until about 1940.

In 1890, the Royal Society of London was shocked when Walter Heape reported how he transferred a fertilized egg from a mother Angora rabbit to a foster mother of the Belgian rabbit line. Other scientists began applying Heape's procedures to other species. By 1956 Whitten succeeded in developing eight-cell mouse embryos to the blastocyst stage *in vitro* in a special culture medium. They then transferred the embryos to many mammal species, including cat, dog, and water buffalo. Improvements in this technique led R. G. Edwards and gynecologist P. Steptoe (1913–1988) to the ultimate achievement in 1978—the birth of the first test-tube baby, healthy, five-pound twelve-ounce Louise Joy Brown.

Researchers who followed were able to study living embryos using the more refined techniques of isolation, transplantation, and tissue culture. The U.S. scientist Ross G. Harrison (1870–1959) studied early organ determination. Hans Spemann (1869–1941) refined the techniques of experimental embryology and carried out systematic studies of development. A master of the art of microdissection, Spemann sought to discover the precise moment when a particular embryonic structure started on the path to differentiation. Using embryonic eggs of the salamander, he and his student Hilda Mangold (1898–1924) grafted the area called the dorsal lip of an unpigmented salamander embryo to the flank of a pigmented host embryo. Three days later a complete secondary embryo appeared—a mosaic of host and donor cells. Because the dorsal lip graft was powerful enough to generate the new embryo, they called it the "organizer region." In 1935 Spemann was awarded the Nobel Prize in Physiology or Medicine for his discovery of the organizer effect in the induction of embryonic development.

In the 1930s embryologists found that cells from the organizer region could start a new embryo, even after they were killed by heating, freezing, or alcohol treatment. These experiments led to the idea that the inducing tissues released something like "magic molecules." Repeated failures to find these molecules led researchers to abandon the idea of organizer regions, but a new biochemical approach to the study of embryology had been established. Developments of the second half of the twentieth century, following the bombshell discovery of DNA, would lead to a new approach, and to the idea of stem cells.

STUDIES OF REGENERATION

The second area of exploration that led to the concept of stem cells was the realm of regeneration. The idea that animals can grow new body parts had been around since the time of Aristotle. An ancient Greek myth told of the multi-headed monster—the hydra—could grow new heads if one was severed. As his second labor, Hercules was commanded to kill the Lernean Hydra, a nine-headed serpent that terrorized the countryside. When Hercules smashed one head, two more would burst out in the place of the destroyed one. It was not a myth that lizards, crabs, cockroaches, and starfishes were observed to grow new body parts, or that a salamander could regrow the same leg many times.

Rene-Antoine Ferchault de Reaumur (1683–1757), one of the great natural philosophers, was probably the first person to study regeneration seriously. He presented a paper on the regeneration of crayfish limbs to the French Academy in 1712 and caused quite a stir with drawings that illustrated how these animals could regenerate parts of their claws.

Abraham Trembly of Geneva, Switzerland (1710–1784), the thirty-year-old tutor of the two sons of Count William Bentinck, worked hard to entertain the minds of his young students. He decided they might be interested in investigating some of the life in a stream with a handheld magnifier. Holding tight to one of the plants was a small bud-like creature. Trembly decided this creature was an animal and began studying it. If he split its head, each area would generate a new head. He called this animal the hydra after the mythological creature that grew two heads when one was severed. He found that if he cut the animal into pieces, each piece would grow a new body, and that the progression followed a pattern of small to large, similar to how an embryo develops. His experiments were the first to document that some animals could generate asexually. However, Trembly never pondered the question of how could the animals' parts could have the power to act like an embryo.

Charles Bonnet (1720–1793), Trembly's cousin, was also interested in regeneration. Studying salamanders, he observed that the creature's eye could regenerate. He also launched a major study of aphids, and was the first to propose the idea that female aphids were able to reproduce without fertilization by the male, a phenomenon called **parthenogenesis.** He presented his research to the French Academy in 1745. Bonnet also coined the term "evolution," used in the biological context of responding to catastrophic events.

Italian scientist Lazarro Spallanzani (1729–1799) was greatly influenced by Bonnet and his studies of invertebrates. He investigated how salamanders can also regrow limbs, tails, and jaws, and confirmed Bonnet's observations that earthworms can regenerate. He also studied vertebrates and was the first to perform the successful artificial insemination of a dog. Probably one of his most notable accomplishments was the debunking of a theory popular at the time—spontaneous generation. This idea held that living things, like flies, came from rotten meat.

Most scientists of this period believed wrongly that inside the body there exist preformed materials. These theorists borrowed certain ideas from the development of embryology, which held that human embryos came from organs preformed in the egg or sperm. In 1838 Germans Mattias Schleiden and Theodor Schwann concluded that the cell is the basic unit of life. Many decades passed before the idea was conceived that groups of cells form tissues. Several years later in 1855, Rudolph Virchow observed that every cell comes from another cell. More years would pass before scientists determined that the hydra has cells that are arranged in two layers, and that the unusual process of regeneration depends on embryonic cells present in the hydra.

From the beginning to the end of the nineteenth century, great strides were made in biology. Microscopes improved, and investigation into cell characteristics expanded. Gregor Mendel (1822–1884), experimenting with plants, formed the basis of the first law of heredity: the law of segregation. This law posits that all hereditary units are in pairs and that genes in a pair separate during division of a cell. Half the sperm or eggs will contain a gene in a pair. Thomas Hunt Morgan (1866–1945) was interested in Mendel's work. Morgan began his research studying regeneration, and coined the terms "morphallaxis" and "epimorphosis" to describe the varied phenomena he observed. Morphallaxis occurs when the body part regenerates but the cells themselves do not appear to grow; epimorphosis occurs when the cells do multiply. The problems of regeneration perplexed Morgan, and he turned his attention to something easier— genetics and the problems of heredity. He later won the Nobel Prize in

Physiology or Medicine for his work in genetics and developmental biology. Morgan may be considered the father of modern genetics.

Regeneration studies may still shed light on stem cell research. In his University of Utah laboratory, Shannon Odelberg is studying the newt's remarkable ability to regenerate limbs, spinal cords, hearts, tails, retinas, lenses, and upper and lower jaws. Scientists in Odelberg's lab in Salt Lake City, Utah, have found that during the initial phase of regeneration, cells in the area of the injury reverse themselves and become stem cells again. Known as dedifferentiation, the process produces cells that will later grow and redifferentiate to form the new part or organ. The process is unique and is not observed in animals that lack regenerative powers, such as mammals. Odelberg's team of scientists are looking for those genes that regulate regeneration and are investigating the possibility of translating them to mammals—even to humans. They are looking in particular for the molecular processes related to the spinal cord, heart, and limbs.

OF MONSTERS AND MICE

One offshoot of research in the nineteenth century was the study of animal formation and monstrosities, which led to an experimental science called teratogeny, or the art of producing monstrosities in animal embryos. In 1822 biological philosopher Etienne Geoffrey Saint-Hilaire published two volumes of the first detailed work completely dedicated to the study of malformations. His son Isadore invented the term "teratology," from the Greek *teratos,* meaning "monster" and *ology,* meaning "study of." Camille Dareste developed the experiments and credited himself with making teratology into the science of teratogeny. He created all the monsters that had been listed in the past and speculated about the possibility of developing some completely new ones. Today the terms have changed to become politically correct. The experiments continue to deal with abnormal and congenital malformations but leave out the word "monstrosity," although Australian sociologist and historian Melinda Cooper (2004) has argued that the field of regenerative medicine and stem cell research is tied to the nineteenth-century tradition of teratology. As science in the century developed, the study of the meaning of disease came into focus. The famous physician Claude Bernard (1813–1878) sought to reduce the incidence of pathology as a variation of the normal equilibrium of the body. But Cooper contends that teratogeny studied form and function, and represented a counterphilosophy pointing in the direction of stem cell research. In other words, study of the unusual leads to understanding of the normal.

Isadore Saint-Hilaire wrote on parasitic monstrosities, or embryonic growths that exist in the mother's uterus or ovary and sprout hair, fatty tissue, teeth, and cartilage, strangely like a normal embryo. What he was describing is a special type of ovarian tumor, coined in 1863 a "teratoma."

These monstrosities have a long medical history. In ancient tablets, pictures of teratomas of the testes and spine of newborns are found. When dissections of corpses became commonplace in the seventeenth century, medical texts—such as one published in 1658—illustrated the teratoma sprouting hair. These phenomena were thought to arise from nightmares or witchcraft; in the nineteenth century, perverse sexuality was theorized as causing them. But Isadore Saint-Hilaire contended they were the product of conception. Thus the history of stem cells can be traced to teratogeny and the experiments that sought to create monsters in animals.

Leroy Stevens and the Jackson Lab

In 1953 Leroy Stevens, a junior researcher at the Jackson Laboratory in Bar Harbor, Maine, was assigned to look for outward signs of cancer in mice that had specific genes. Dr. Clarence Cook Little established the Jackson Lab in 1929 to study and produce mice for research. A major tobacco company had awarded a grant to the laboratory for a study the company hoped would prove that cigarette paper, not tobacco, causes cancer. After exposure to large amounts of cigarette ingredients, Stevens noticed some of the mice had large growths in the testicles, possibly indicating a teratoma. Little encouraged Stevens, and was convinced he had found something important. Dissecting the mouse, Stevens found a unique combination of cells that did not belong there. Twitching and pulsating cells, more like those found in cardiac muscle, were present along with a confusing variety of other cells. Calling this strain "mouse 129," Stevens autopsied hundreds of them and found that many had the same teratomas. This indicated that somewhere in the line was a defective gene. But the teratoma proved to be more important. The teratoma had both undifferentiated and differentiated cells. In some of the more advanced specimens, more than 14 different types of differentiated mature cells were found, including hair, bone, intestine, blood, and others. The critical leap came when Jackson Lab scientists recognized that the early, or precursor, cells that caused cancer closely resembled the cells in the embryo. Stevens implanted these early embryo cells that included cells in the ICM into testes of adult mice. Just as he expected, teratomas formed. He called the ICM cells "pluripotent embryonic stem cells," a term that is now familiar. But these cells did cause cancer and were referred to as **embryonal carcinoma cells (ECCs).** EC cells were very difficult to develop because their chromosomes were unstable.

Barry Pierce, on the faculty at the University of Michigan, added another piece to the puzzle. In 1964 he demonstrated that single undifferentiated cells isolated from one of the mouse teratomas and injected into normal mice could cause tumors that had tissues of all three major germ layers. Using light microscopy, he found both undifferentiated malignant cells interspersed with disorganized adult somatic cells at various stages of differentiation. He hypothesized that most cancers contain a pool of malignant stem cells and benign noncancerous cells. The progeny of some of the malignant tumor cells could differentiate into nonmalignant cells. In effect, he proposed that a malignant cell could become benign, an idea that challenged the dogma of the day—once a cancer cell, always a cancer cell. His work was met with skepticism because teratomas were considered oddities among cancers. However, in 1971, Pierce and Carol Wallace found similar differentiated and undifferentiated stem cells in squamous cell carcinomas, a type of skin cancer.

In 1981, Gail R. Martin and a team of scientists isolated ESCs that had stable chromosomes and did not cause cancer. These mouse ESCs became the foundation of **knockout technology,** a system for the creation of laboratory animals with certain kinds of genetic makeup.

In England in the 1980s, investigators attempted to extract stem cells from human embryos and were interested in learning what stem cells could teach them about early development. In 1987 Christopher Graham at Oxford set out to study the biological or genetic factors in human embryos that regulate their potent cells. At that time the therapeutic value of stem cells had not occurred to the investigators.

The history of adult stem cells began in the 1960s. Researchers discovered that the bone marrow contains at least two kinds of stem cells. One kind—hematopoietic cells—forms all types of blood cells. A second type—bone marrow stromal cells—is a mixed population of the cells that generate bone, cartilage, and fibrous connective tissue. Also in the 1960s, scientists studying rats found two regions of the brain that have dividing cells, which become nerve cells. However, it was not until the 1990s that scientists agreed that the brain contains stem cells.

The study of stem cell research is founded in the three historical fields of reproductive biology, regeneration studies, and studies of teratomas, the rare cancerous tumors. With the great technological progress of the twentieth century have emerged regenerative medicine, stem cell research, and gene therapy. However, the science is still in its infancy with many historical questions a long way from being answered.

CHAPTER 3

Current Stem Cell Research Since 1990

The second half of the twentieth century exploded with technology for studying biology. The struggle to map the genome, accomplished in 2000, gave impetus to the tools of microscopy, microdissection, and chemical media for growth of cells. It had been nearly 30 years since Leroy Stevens's initial discovery at the Jackson Lab, with scientists cloistered behind laboratory walls, determinedly following the motto, never give up. The isolation of embryonic stem cells was a watershed discovery and occurred simultaneously in two laboratories. One team, from the Johns Hopkins University School of Medicine in Baltimore, harvested stem cells from aborted fetuses. A second team, from the Wisconsin Regional Primate Research Center in Madison, used leftover blastocysts from fertility clinics.

In the mid-1990s investigators were having trouble isolating the stem cells from the embryos. Using embryos left over from in vitro fertilization (IVF) was a problem. The good embryos were used for implantation, leaving the inferior ones to be placed in cold storage. The effect on cells of the periods of freezing was unknown.

JOHNS HOPKINS UNIVERSITY SCHOOL OF MEDICINE

In 1995 John Gearhart at Johns Hopkins decided to investigate a source of embryos other than frozen castoffs. He would isolate the precursor to egg or sperm—called primordial germ cells (PGC)—from the gonads of an aborted 8- to 12-week-old fetus. He surmised that these cells from the early germ cell would be as pluripotent as the ones in the embryo. Although unproven, his guess was rational because it is the egg and sperm that create new human beings.

Gearhart had studied Stevens's famous mice, and absorbed the burgeoning knowledge of the field of embryology. Since the 1950s, the science of embryology was slowly evolving into the new science of developmental biology, a discipline that recognizes that development continues beyond the embryo. Gearhart inherited maps that trace the origins of specific cells in the embryo to a specific tissue pathway. In addition, he had a background in plant genetics and was familiar with experiments in which mature plant cells had been taken apart (i.e., had been dedifferentiated) using a certain culture medium. His dream was to take mature plant cells, render them to the totipotent stage in the right culture, and make a new plant. But his life took a new path when he accepted a position in a laboratory in Philadelphia with a focus on cloning and on carcinoma stem cells.

By chance, Gearhart's niche in medicine became the study of a mammal's first weeks of development and solving the problems that arise during this process. In 1979 Johns Hopkins hired him to teach embryology and research the embryogenesis of mammals. By the early 1990s Gearhart had become a premier investigator of a Down-like syndrome in mice, but wanted to expand his research beyond mice. Now that stem cells had been isolated from mouse embryos, Gearhart was riveted to the possibility of extending this knowledge to human embryos. He had no philosophical objection to the practice of abortion and supported the right of a woman to choose to end her unwanted pregnancy. He did not appreciate the waste of the discarded fetus after abortion and believed it unethical to throw the issue away.

Gearhart approached Johns Hopkins's **Institutional Review Board (IRB)** to inquire into research on human embryos. The university investigational review that followed lasted three years—from 1993 to 1996—before approving his research proposal. In 1996 Gearhart and graduate student Michael Shamblott isolated a germ cell about the size of a tiny bit of rice, but this find was short-lived: the cell did not divide. Eventually they concocted a growth factor culture medium that would allow embryonic germ cells to live longer periods of time.

From the Roslin Institute in Edinburgh, Scotland, on February 23, 1997, came an announcement that shook the world and also gave encouragement to embryonic cell researchers. Ian Wilmut and colleagues had cloned a sheep they named Dolly. The scientists injected an egg cell with the nucleus of a mammary gland cell that contained the mother's genetic information. Returning to the totipotent stage, the egg developed into Dolly the sheep. Dolly and other successful clones garnered lots of attention, with some media outlets billing the event as something out of *Brave New World,* the 1932 novel by Aldous Huxley that tells of a world where children are genetically engineered and programmed for their role in society. Gearhart required the scientists in his laboratory to view the film version of the novel and be prepared for the tough questions about their research that would follow. In the November 10, 1998, issue of the *Proceedings of the National Academy of Science,* Gearhart and team announced they had gathered evidence substantiating that fetal cells could generate the three germ layers endoderm, ectoderm, and mesoderm, and keep on growing.

WISCONSIN PRIMATE RESEARCH CENTER

James Thomson arrived at Madison, Wisconsin, in 1991 to work at the University of Wisconsin. He had earned doctorates in veterinary medicine and molecular biology at the University of Pennsylvania and was attracted to the idea of capturing the stem cells of mouse embryos. He had studied at several prestigious primate centers. His challenge at Madison was to capture stem cells from rhesus monkeys, a difficult task because the female reproductive organs of this species are very complex. Using unique devices he created, he reported the first embryonic stem cells from a nonhuman primate in November 1995. He and others expected that human embryo cells could be their next challenge.

Since the 1973 U.S. Supreme Court decision in *Roe v. Wade* that made abortion legal for women up to the point of viability, the human embryo and fetus had become a hot political topic. In 1988 President Ronald Reagan prohibited spending federal funds for research involving fetal tissue from induced abortions, although private funds could still be used. Bill Clinton lifted the ban in January 1993. As many as 1.5 million fetuses were aborted each year in the early 1990s, and there was growing concern that these fetuses might be grown and aborted for financial gain. Thousands of embryos from in vitro fertilization were stored in freezers.

Thomson was motivated to pursue the human stem cell because the university operated its own IVF clinic. He surmised that some couples, clients of the clinic, may be willing to part with their unused stored embryos if they realized the possibilities of future breakthroughs in medicine. However, funding would be a hurdle. He applied to the Wisconsin Alumni Research Foundation, which promptly rejected his project. In 1995 Thomson met Michael West, the entrepreneur who founded the biotechnology firm, Geron. Geron's mission is to study the cellular basis of aging and to design drugs to stop the process. West offered to fund human stem cell research in exchange for a license to patent the rhesus monkey embryonic stem (ES) cells for research on aging at Geron.

The next hurdle would be getting the project approved by the university's 24-member Health Sciences Human Subject Committee. Such review boards operate at all institutions where research on human subjects is conducted, to ensure it is carried out in an ethical manner and with the informed consent of the parties involved. After long and heated debate, the board gave Thomson the go-ahead to accept funds to pursue stem cells from IVF embryos. Geron's scientists would be able to use the cells of rhesus monkeys to analyze the enzyme **telomerase,** which keeps the **telomere** (i.e., the end of the cell) long and healthy.

Thomson's research did not enjoy smooth sailing. The IVF embryos that were not transferred to the women were frozen right after they were made. If a woman did not become pregnant, one of her reserve embryos would be thawed, grown to day two or three, and then implanted in the uterus. But it was not possible to grow the egg to day five or six, the blastocyst stage when the mass of stem cells is optimal. Thomson collaborated with IVF lab director Jeffrey Jones to find a culture that would sustain the cells. Studying the amino acids that make up the fallopian tube and the uterus, the pair made a medium that would allow the stem cells to grow to the inner cell mass. On November 6, 1998, Thomson's research on the isolation and culturing of human embryonic stem cells appeared in the journal *Science.* The private, not-for-profit WiCell Research Institute was formed to distribute stem cells for basic stem cell research. In the face of political controversy, the University of Wisconsin Board of Regents adopted a resolution to support research using human stem cells on March 9, 2001.

THE STORY OF ADULT STEM CELLS

In the 1970s researchers working with mice began to uncover the fact that stem cells were found in other organs of the body. Ernest McCullough and James Till found evidence of a blood-making stem cell in adult mice. Muscle cells were found to build muscle fiber, and cells in the intestine were found to be able to refurbish the intestinal lining. In 1968 Joseph Altman, scanning the brains of young rats, found what he thought were new nerve cells. When grown in a petri dish, the neural stem cells changed into three main cells—neurons, astrocytes, and oligodendrocytes. In 1998 scientists at the Salk Institute in California and at

Sahlgrenska University in Sweden found that human stem cells did lead to regeneration of certain cells in the brain. From several arenas, adult stem cells were considered a possible source. This idea was attractive because it avoided many of the ethical questions that plagued research based on embryonic stem cells.

Adult stem cells from bone marrow have been widely used with chemotherapy to treat leukemia. After killing the cancer cells, oncologists inject into the bloodstream stem cells that migrate to areas of the body where they are needed to regenerate the immune system. The success of this model predicts future success with many diseases. Chapters 5, 6, and 7 discuss specific research in detail.

THE MOVE TO CLINICAL MEDICINE

Stem cells challenged Ariff Bongso as a doctoral student at Ontario Veterinary College. Born in Ceylon (now Sri Lanka) of a Dutch mother and Sri Lankan Muslim father, he developed a passion for mammalian embryos and studied a wide range of embryos, from cow to water buffalo. He sought to identify the sex of the embryo from the earliest stages, an accomplishment that would aid in beef and milk production efficiency. Bongso soon made the leap from the study of animal embryos to the study of human ones in England, where he was introduced to in vitro fertilization. In 1983 he joined a team of fertility researchers who were responsible for Asia's first test-tube baby and who helped make Singapore a center for IVF in South Asia.

In 1986 Bongso went to work at the National University of Singapore, where he was provided an environment of discipline, transparency, and financial support, and accomplished many firsts in the IVF field. In 1989 he produced the world's first micromanipulation baby. In this process sperm from a male with a very low sperm count are injected under the shells of eggs to fertilize them. Bongso helped develop a novel in vitro system called coculture in which embryos are grown on a bed of human fallopian tube cells. Growing the cells on human tissue frees the embryo from the mouse media (i.e., from *xeno,* or foreign, cultures). In 1992 Bongso led a team that produced the world's first babies that were implanted after their first five-day, or blastocyst, stage of development. In 1997 the first babies were grown in this culture that allows the entire shell of the embryo to be removed before transfer to assist implantation in older women. Coculture also enables doctors to fertilize many eggs and freeze them, against the chance the first attempt does not succeed.

Coculture became an important technique that quietly led to unlocking the secrets of the mysterious cells of the human embryo. In 1994 Bongso became the first to isolate stem cells from a five-day-old embryo. He documented that these cells could transform themselves into any cell in the human body. His research appeared in the *Human Reproduction* journal, published by the Oxford University Press.

On August 5, 2002 Bongso announced that his team had successfully grown a human embryonic stem cell (hESC) line entirely without mouse cells. The new cell line had been grown on human feeder cells and cell nutrients. Realizing the importance of making the cells available to scientists for their research, Bongso approached the Singaporean government, which handsomely funded his spin-off company, Embryonic Stem Cell International. Other investors included Next Wave Singapore and a private group of Australian businesspersons.

Bongso believes that applied stem cell research is critical. The ability to use these lines without exposure to mouse cells eliminates the potential risk of pathogens transferring from animal to human embryonic cells. In 2002 all 78 existing stem cell lines in the United States were grown on animal or mouse feeder cell layers, which eliminates their use for human trials. The U.S. Food and Drug Administration has set the gold standard for stem cells grown for human therapeutics: they must be animal-free.

Bongso is also pursuing safer storage systems for stem cell lines. The current practice of storing the cells in open plastic straws and freezing them in liquid nitrogen is not ideal. A virus could possibly be lurking that would contaminate the cells. Bongso is developing an electronic system that promises to reduce the incidence of contamination.

Now focusing his energies on unlocking cells' genetic secrets, Bongso has launched into determining which genes are responsible for instructions for developing the 210 tissue cells. From fertilization to pregnancy, genes are continually being switched off and on, telling stem cells whether to become a liver, heart, or bone cell. Having lost his mother to cancer and his father to hemorrhagic stroke, Bongso fervently believes the field of regenerative medicine holds promise for those suffering with a variety of diseases.

In Massachusetts, seven Harvard schools, seven teaching hospitals, and more than 100 researchers and scientists have come together to form the Harvard Stem Cell Institute (HSCI). The goal of the institute is to use stem cells to help the 150 million people who are living with five types of organ and tissue failure. Institute codirector Douglas Melton established HSCI to consolidate research and disseminate information to sites that are already engaged in stem cell research. Their goal is to move from the laboratory bench to the bedside, and make a difference in human health.

THERAPEUTIC CLONING

Therapeutic cloning is the development of embryos for use in treating illnesses. Rudolf Jaenisch, a founding member of the Whitehead Institute in Cambridge, Massachusetts, demonstrated in the 1970s that foreign

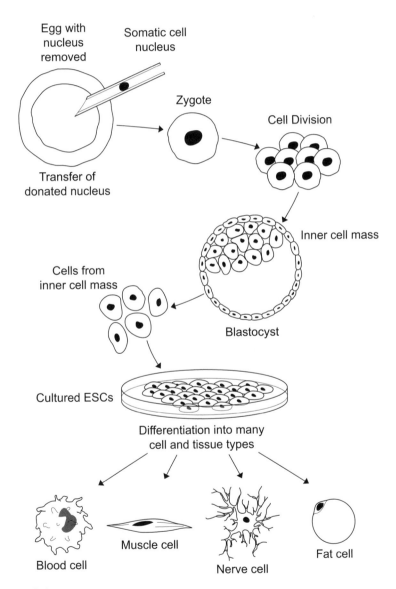

Figure 3.1
Somatic cell nuclear transfer. (Illustration by Jeff Dixon.)

DNA could be inserted into the DNA of early mouse embryos, and that the offspring would carry foreign genes in all their tissues. Later he created the first transgenic mice by introducing leukemia DNA sequences into the mouse genome. The offspring of these mice carried the DNA.

Jaenisch is a leader in the field of **therapeutic cloning** (i.e., therapeutic nuclear transfer). In this process the genetic information of a cell is transplanted into an unfertilized egg from which the DNA has been removed, as shown in Figure 3.1. When the egg is placed in a petri dish, a blastocyst forms, from which stem cells can be taken. The procedure has been performed only in mice although it is also applicable to humans. Using a technique called altered nuclear transfer, Jaenisch has been able to isolate stem cells without harming a viable embryo. He is striving to understand the biological mechanisms that affect how genetic information is converted into cell structures without altering the genes in the process. This is called epigenetic regulation of gene expression. Jaenisch's laboratory is also investigating epigenetic mechanisms for certain types of cancer, and for brain development in conditions like Rett syndrome.

George P. Dailey, a pediatrician at the Children's Hospital in Boston, is another expert in therapeutic cloning. He works in both the research lab and the clinic, but views stem cell research as the discipline that will translate from lab bench to bedside. Therapeutic cloning is not reproductive cloning, but cloning that uses cells only for therapeutic purposes. In fact, Jaenisch is opposed to human reproductive cloning, which involves placement of the cloned egg into the uterus.

The last decade of the twentieth century saw great developments in the science of stem cell research, where progress exploded in both private and public laboratories. Overcoming the problem of cell growth without contamination is a practical challenge, and ethical objections and questions have led to the imposition of government regulations. Section Two discusses the ethics of stem cell research and efforts to regulate it.

CHAPTER 4

Taking Care: Growing and Maintaining Embryonic Stem Cells

Myrna Watkins, Coordinator of Health, Wellness, and Physical Education for the Marion County, Florida, school district, happened to pick up a brochure about cord blood. It touted the benefits of collecting and storing the blood from a new baby's umbilical cord as a great gift to give a child or grandchild. Her daughter Francie was expecting in February, and as a person who likes to be on the cutting edge, Myrna decided this would be a unique gift for her grandchild. Francie, who had the same mind-set, also thought that it would be a great idea. Her husband agreed. His family, however, disapproved. They thought that performing such a procedure would be playing God.

When her daughter went into labor early, Myrna rushed to Indiana for the birth. She had not had time to plan the gift and stayed on the phone for hours while Francie was in labor, trying to locate someone who knew about collecting cord blood. Finally, Myrna called Jewish Hospital in Louisville, Kentucky, which contacted Viacord. The Viacord representatives were there in two hours and ten minutes—in time for the birth of Myrna's grandchild. However, Myrna was later informed that cord blood can be collected for as long as several hours after birth. In 2001 Myrna paid $1,000 for the collection; she pays $100 per year for storage. She says she has no reason not to believe that some day in the future one of the siblings or other family members may need the blood; it was a good investment. Myrna admits she does not know much about stem cell research, and at times, the thought does go through her mind that her gift may have been premature. But, when she reads about the burgeoning technological advances, she knows that stem cell–based therapy is the wave of the future. Her gift is insurance.

GROWING STEM CELLS

Like Myrna, many people have no idea what happens in stem cell research. They do not realize what a complicated and tedious process it is. This chapter looks at how stem cells are prepared for use in the laboratory and how scientists must treat them tenderly, like newborn infants.

Hours of rigorous training go into learning how to extract and grow approved stem cells. One place scientists go to study the intricate laboratory techniques is the WiCell center in Madison, Wisconsin. Armed with blue latex gloves and forceps, here the scientist-student will spend approximately four hours dissecting a pregnant mouse, taking out the tiny uterus and locating the embryos, which look like pods full of small red peas. The scientists clean the embryos and break them apart until they look like red mashed potatoes. Now ready to grow in a petri dish, this luxurious bed of mouse cells is the future home to a few human embryonic cells. However, the challenge is to pamper the mouse cells with just the right nutrients to help them divide properly and not become crowded. If a new layer of nutrients is not provided every two weeks, the mouse cells will die.

After the beds are prepared, the questions of stem cells and their sources arise. Three simple but hard-to-answer questions need to be addressed in considering in vitro differentiated cells to replace in vivo tissue:

- Which cells should be used and how to obtain them?
- Where do the cells go after they are injected into the patient?
- What do they do once they are in the body?

These questions, along with experiment design, must be considered in detail using animal models.

Sources for stem cells include bone marrow–derived cells, peripheral derived blood cells, embryonic stem cells, amniotic blood cells, cord blood cells, muscle-derived cells, parthenogenetic stem cells, fused stem cells, and therapeutic cloning.

SOURCES OF STEM CELLS

Bone Marrow–Derived Stem Cells

Bone marrow appears to contain three types of stem cell populations: hematopoietic (hSCs), **endothelial progenitor,** and **mesenchymal.** The hSCs produce all types of blood cells in the body. Endothelial progenitor cells differentiate into endothelial flat cells that line the blood and lymphatic vessels, the heart, and various other body cavities. Mesenchymal cells, a network of cells derived from the embryonic mesoderm, give rise to connective tissues and other parts of the cardiovascular system. Each of these kinds of stem cells can be isolated from adult bone marrow and appear to have the potential for multiple lineages of differentiation.

Peripheral Blood–Derived Stem Cells

Cells isolated from adult human peripheral blood have been shown to differentiate into nonhematopoietic tissues, such as epithelial cells of the gastrointestinal tract and skin.

Embryonic Stem Cells

Embryonic stem cells (ESCs), embryonic germinal cells (EGCs), and embryonic carcinoma cells (ECCs) are all human pluripotent stem cells. They are all capable of self-renewal, a property that other, more differentiated cells have lost. However, each of these cells differs in its **karyotype** (i.e., the photomicrograph of the nucleus of the individual cell). For example, ECCs have an excess of chromosomes. Telomerase, an enzyme that controls chromosome length, is very active in all of these cell types. Telomeres are located at the ends of chromosomes; the enzyme telomerase replaces them after each round of cell division to prevent shortening of the chromosomes. A large number of transcription factors—a wide assortment of proteins needed to initiate or regulate transcription of the copying of a DNA sequence into RNA—are also present in each of these cells.

Embryonic stem cells (ESCs) are the most primitive of all populations of stem cells. They develop as part of the inner cell mass of the human blastocyst at day five after fertilization. At such an early stage, this type of stem cell has vast development potential and can give rise to cells of all three embryonic germ layers. When cultured in appropriate media and culture conditions, ESCs can undergo an unlimited number of doublings and retain the capacity to differentiate into any cell type. ESCs are currently not approved for human implantation because of the immunosuppression requirements necessary to avoid rejection of the transplanted cells and development of teratomas.

EGCs give rise to **embryoid bodies,** which contain both differentiated and nondifferentiated cells. Embryoid bodies are collections of hundreds of cells that resemble early embryos and are produced by growing the germ cells in the presence of retinoic acid. These cells are found in the gonadal ridge of the embryo or fetus and normally develop into mature gametes of sperm and eggs when the organism is fully developed.

Essential requirements for transplantation of human ESCs and EGCs are:

- Quality control of the cell expansion process
- Generation of sufficient quantities of cells
- Induction in the host of tolerance to grafted cells

Concerns have been raised about the transplantability of human cells derived in vitro from stem cells. Chromosomal abnormalities have been observed in different studies and appear most frequently in chromosomes 2, 12, and 1.

Amniotic Fluid as a Source

Amniotic fluid has been used for screening developmental and genetic diseases for more than 70 years. In 1930 the first reported **amniocentesis** attempted to connect the examination of cell concentration, count, and phenotypes with the sex and health of the baby. In amniocentesis a large needle is inserted into the mother's abdominal region to draw out some of the fluid. Karyotyping then shows a systematized array of metaphase chromosomes. By analyzing these chromosomes, scientists have found that amniotic fluid, as well as the later development of ultrasound-guided amniocentesis, provides reliable diagnostic markers, including fetoprotein.

However, the fluid may be a source of undifferentiated cells as well as those that have differentiated into the three germ cell layers. Ultrasound detects the amniotic sac at about 10 weeks and harvesting the cells would take place at around 16 weeks. Paolo De Coppi and co-authors (2006) believe that pluripotent progenitor cells—parent cells that give rise to a distinct cell lineage by a series of cell divisions—isolated from amniotic fluid present an exciting possibility for stem cell biology and regenerative medicine. Isolated cells have developed into liver, muscle, nerve, bone, fat, and skin.

Amniotic fluid cells may have a better possibility for expansion than adult stem cells. These progenitor cells can be cryopreserved for future use and have considerable advantages. They easily differentiate into specific cell lineages, do not need feeder layers to grow, and do not require the sacrifice of human embryos. Amniotic fluid cells represent a great source for therapeutic application where large numbers of cells are needed. They are similar to embryonic stem cells in the following ways:

- They can differentiate into three germ layers.
- They express common markers.

- They preserve their telomere length. (A telomere is a specialized nucleic acid structure at the ends of chromosomes.)

These cells were recently discovered, and a great deal of work remains to be done on their characterization and use. Initial results have been promising, according to De Coppi and co-authors.

Cord Blood

Blood from the umbilical cord is another promising source of stem cells. In October 1989 cord blood was used to cure the fatal condition Fanconi anemia. The cord blood was taken from a female sibling whose blood type matched the male recipient's. Dr. Hal Broxmeyer, Distinguished Professor of Medicine at Indiana University, first used cord blood transplantation as a proof-of-principle treatment, based on the use of a substance previously considered waste material.

Since 1989 more than 5,000 individuals with various malignant and genetic disorders have received transplants from umbilical cord blood of hematopoietic stem cells—those that can make more of themselves and give rise to blood-forming tissue—and progenitor cells. The transplantation works in both children and adults, but it has been used mainly in children because of the apparently limited number of stem-progenitor cells in a single cord blood collection. Since the initial clinical studies, cord blood banks have been developed worldwide, thereby allowing the expansion of cord blood transplantation from related to unrelated donors.

CorCell, like Viacord, the company described in the introduction to this chapter, stores umbilical cord blood. Company representatives emphasize the absence of risk and pain to mother and baby when explaining the cord blood collection process. In addition to being painless, the use of cord blood also poses a lower risk of post-transplant **graft-versus-host disease (GVHD)** than other types of blood stem cell transplantation. Cord blood allows for perfect matches of **human leukocyte antigen (HLA)** type. HLAs are proteins on the white blood cells that can cause rejection if a match is not close enough. Testing determines whether a patient is a suitable stem cell donor.

Muscle-Derived Cells

Skeletal muscle, unlike other types of muscle, is able to regenerate and repair itself after injury due to the presence of immature satellite cells, or myoblasts. They are quiet in normal skeletal muscle but, upon injury, enter the cycle.

Parthenogenetic Stem Cells

Can an egg develop into an embryo without being fertilized by a sperm? Some scientists are investigating a process that takes place in aphids, bees, ants, and in some instances, frogs. Parthenogenesis is derived from the Greek words for "virgin birth." Charles Bonnet, an eighteenth-century investigator, first discovered the phenomenon. Later, Jacques Loeb (1859–1924) demonstrated the first clear case of parthenogenesis when he pricked unfertilized eggs with a needle and found that normal embryonic development occurred. In 1936 Gregory Pincus activated rabbit's eggs by varying temperature and chemical agents. Subsequently, others have investigated molecular events that have led to oocyte activation in invertebrates, amphibians, and mice.

Recently, parthenogenesis has received attention for its potential use in the production of stem cells. In 1983 M. H. Kaufman showed that pluripotency is a possibility in mouse cells. Although stem cell lines have been produced in nonhuman primates, no human parthenogenetic model has been advanced. Using unfertilized human eggs may be less controversial. They may also have the advantage of being homozygous, providing a broader match than mesenchymal human cells. This technique is promising for cell-based therapies for a variety of disorders including Parkinson's disease, Alzheimer's disease, and diabetes.

Fused Stem Cells

In August 2005 Harvard scientists announced that they had created cells similar to human embryonic stem cells without destroying embryos: a major step toward defusing the central objection to stem cell research. They fused a human skin cell with an embryonic stem cell, which produced a hybrid that looked and acted like a stem cell. One advantage to this cell fusion technique is that it allows stem cells to be tailor-made for patients. Kevin Eggan, the chief investigator among the Harvard scientists, noted that with its flaws and inefficiencies, this technology is not yet "ready for prime time," although it is a possible step toward defusing the controversy over the use of embryonic stem cells. This process is discussed in Chapter 13.

THERAPEUTIC CLONING

In 2002 Advanced Cell Technology reported that it had grown kidneys from cloned cow embryos. The purpose was to demonstrate that cloned animals and subsequent embryos could be a histocompatible source of stem cells. Attempting to grow the kidney in culture, Robert Lanza and colleagues cloned cows from ear epithelium and allowed the embryo to reach the early fetal stage. They then cultured the cells on a collagen-coated renal bed to grow the artificial organ, known as an embryoid kidney. They implanted the embryoid kidney under the skin of the same adult cow that had produced the clones. This technology is in its early experimental stage—a great deal of work remains to be completed before questions about it are answered.

Human patients have very poor options when it comes to treating kidney disorders:

- They may live on kidney dialysis for the rest of their lives.
- They may have a kidney transplant and take immunosuppressants for the remainder of their lives.
- They may try therapeutic cloning.

In therapeutic cloning, doctors harvest a patient's stem cells and then implant them back into the patient. Unfortunately, society is not ready for the idea of therapeutic cloning.

FACING REJECTION

Stem cells from the sources detailed above must be injected into a patient to make necessary repairs. The procedure, like an organ transplant, must deal with the immune system. One of the stumbling blocks to any stem cell transplant is finding a matching donor. Matching refers to human leukocyte antigen (HLA) proteins that cover cell surfaces. A person's immune system recognizes these as foreign or belonging to an outsider. For a transplant to be successful, the HLAs must be very similar.

The source of the transplant provides the name. An **autograft** is a transplant of tissue from one part of an individual to some area of the same person. The term **autologous** also describes this procedure. The term **allograft** involves moving tissue from one individual and transplanting that tissue into another, unrelated individual. The proposed transplantation of human embryonic cells into patients suffering with Alzheimer's disease is an example of an allograft, or allogeneic, transplant. **Xenografts** are transplanted from one species to another. For example, transplanting the heart of a pig into a human is a xenograft.

Although autografts do not invoke immune reactions, allografts and xenografts do, and can lead to the serious condition of graft-versus-host disease (GVHD). To avoid GVHD, patients must take strong immunosuppressants like cyclosporin or tacrolimus to kill the immune cells.

GROWING AND MAINTAINING CELLS

Embryonic Cells

Growing and maintaining embryonic stem cells can be likened to taking care of a premature newborn infant—but it's even more complicated. The preemie must be kept in an isolette and watched every moment. An extraordinary level of care is also essential to the survival of ESCs. Both processes are challenging.

Cells grown in the laboratory are known as a cell culture. When scientists determine what they want given cells to become, they have determined **cell fate.** According to their goals for making stem cells become other specific cells, scientists follow procedures that will determine the end product. Different procedures and growth materials affect the cells' outcome, or the cell fate.

Irina Klimanskaya and Jill McMahon (2006) describe the process used in their laboratory. The initial steps for obtaining the cells are conducted under a stereoscopic or dissecting microscope. These microscopes have binocular eyepieces and can project into the third dimension. The microscopes must be fitted with heated stages because the scientists must keep the embryos and the dishes at 37 degrees C. The dissecting microscope must be used under a special hood because the culture is vulnerable to contamination during this time, Under the stereoscope, the colonies are mechanically dispersed. Quality assurance here is very important, and consistent growth conditions are maintained and checked daily with extensive checklists. For example, the temperature must be kept at 37 degrees C, carbon dioxide levels must be 5.0 percent, and the humidity must be kept greater than 90 percent. When expanding for new lines, two incubators are used and are tested with growing mouse embryos. The culture is split between the two incubators as a precaution against any problems that may arise. Incubator doors are seldom opened.

Stem cells must be worked with under conditions even more sterile than required by standard laboratory procedures. Extra precautions are taken because of the limited number of specimens, the labor-intensive nature of the procedures, the team effort involved, and the long period of time required to start a new line. The lines are grown in a petri dish on a **culture medium,** also called a feeder layer. This layer coats the inner surface of the dish and is made of embryonic mouse cells or primary mouse embryo fibroblasts (PMEF) that have been treated so that they will not divide. The reason for having these mouse cells in the culture dish is to give the ICM a sticky surface and provide nutrients for the culture medium. Companies that make the media ship it presterilized directly to the research centers. For safety reasons, however, labs sterilize it again in an autoclave.

The scientists melt an area of a glass tube in a flame until it becomes red-hot and then quickly pull it to make a fine tube. They break the glass at an angle so the end looks like a fine hypodermic needle. Then they place a rubber tube and a suction device on the other end of the tube and begin chopping off and gently sucking in each separated piece of the cell mass into the tube. Mouth suction gives the user more control. They gently blow out pieces of ICM onto the same or another plate.

Over the course of several days, the ICM begins to proliferate and crowd the culture dish. When the embryo is ready for immunosurgery, an acidic solution called Tyrode's solution removes the outer membrane or zona pellucida. Next, a rabbit's anti-human red blood cell antibody binds to the trophoderm, but hopefully not to the ICM. Again the ICM is sucked through a narrow capillary tube and put on a PMEF for further growth and dispersion. Trypsin is added to the colony and, after five days of growth, the colony is transferred to a fresh plate of PMEF. This process of subculturing or replating is repeated many times over many months. After six months, the original 30 or so cells yield millions of embryonic stem cells. The cells are then ready for freezing in dimethyl sulfur oxide (DMSO) and put into cryovials labeled with the line, passage number, and date. The specimen is put in liquid nitrogen at –80 degrees C.

Embryonic cells that have proliferated in culture for more than six months are pluripotent and appear genetically normal—a stem cell line has been created. Throughout the proliferating procedures, cells are tested to see whether they possess the fundamental properties of stem cells, a process called characterization.

In 1998 James Thomson's group collected cells from five-day-old blastocysts obtained from in vitro fertilization clinics. They began with 36 embryos, but only 14 reached the stage of blastocyst. Thomson isolated the inner cell mass from these embryos, using it to establish five human ESC lines: H1, H7, H9, H13, and H14. The medium for growth had been a huge problem for this team, but the development of feeder cells from mice allowed the ESC to grow for two weeks. They were then transferred to plates without the cells and continued to divide without differentiation for six months and were able to form teratomas in mice. Cell line H9 went on to proliferate for more than two years and is used for research throughout the world.

John Gearhart, whose research at Johns Hopkins is described in Chapter 3, used embryonic germ cells collected from the gonadal ridge of a 12-week-old fetus. After 3 weeks, the growth was similar to that of the ESC. He had a similar culture condition except he added a cytokine called the leukemia inhibitory factor (LIF).

The two scientists were stalled in their pursuit of isolating stem cells because they could not find the proper culture medium for growth. The mouse embryo feeder layer—and, later, the fetal calf serum (FCS)—solved the immediate problem, although they did have some major drawbacks. Recently, scientists have begun to devise other ways of growing embryonic stem cells without the mouse feeder layers, thereby reducing the risk of viruses and other macromolecules. To date, two different protocols cultivate in serum-free conditions but still rely on feeder cells. For example, Holly Young and her co-authors (2006) reported a feeder-free culture that maintains hES on Matrigel or laminin-coated plates conditioned with mouse embryo cells. The future challenge is to identify factors that feeder cells release and synthesize.

Unfortunately, the ICM dies when it is removed from a blastocyst. Permission must be granted by the parents in either case before the embryo can be used for research. Adult stem cells provide some relief in the ethical debate. Scientists in many laboratories are trying to find ways to grow adult stem cells in various cell culture media and manipulate them for use in treating injury or disease.

Most available stem cell lines, including those approved for U.S. federal funding, were either generated or grown on animal feeder cells, the nourishing scaffolding often used to support stem cells. Scientists were concerned that animal products could pass viruses or other contaminants to the cells. In March 2005, Robert Lanza and his colleagues at Advanced Cell Technology announced that they had derived a new stem cell line free of any animal cells or serum. They extracted stem cells from a human embryo and grew them on a specially created sterile protein matrix. The cells maintained their ability to grow into different types of tissues, even after six months in the undifferentiated state.

Factors for Differentiating

When the cells are nurtured and collected, the work has only just begun. To determine what the cells will become and how to get them to their final destination is tedious and painstaking. Finding the right conditions that will direct the stem cell to become a particular kind of cell is a process of trial and error. Again, experiments with mouse cells have led the way. The cells that have been isolated from the embryo-like bodies are now replated to form a monolayer of cells. Selecting the growth media is educated guess work. Conditions include: (1) exposing the stem cells to certain growth factors (i.e., to substances that have been isolated and are known to promote growth); (2) exposing them to certain hormones, such as insulin; and (3) injection into mice.

Growth factors are an important part of the process. In 1986 Drs. Rita Levi-Montalcini and Stanley Cohen won the Nobel Prize in Physiology or Medicine for discovering nerve growth factor (NGF), a factor that influences neuronal development in the embryo, and epidermal growth factor (EGF), which is used in treating burns and in stem cell research. Many growth factors are proteins that bind to a special kind of cell protein and function like an enzyme that can **phosphorylate** or activate other proteins. Phosphorylation is a process that acts like a switch to turn on certain processes.

Two other growth factors that aid in differentiation are leukemia inhibitory factor (LIF) and retinoic acid. LIF, expressed in embryonic trophoblasts (the part that forms the placenta), plays an important part in the process of implantation. Retinoic acid, closely related to vitamin A, activates gene expression.

Conditions for growing specific cell types from stem cells include:

- Embryo cell lines can produce epithelial cells or neurons (nerve cells) when exposed to epidermal growth factor (EGF) or nerve growth factor (NGF).
- Embryo cell lines can produce bone, cartilage, smooth muscle, and striated muscle when injected into mice with leukemia inhibitory factor (LIF).
- Stem cells from bone marrow may produce red and white blood cells when injected into mice.
- Stem cells from bone marrow when treated with transforming growth factor (TGF) may produce adipocytes or fat cells.

The process may be quite unpredictable. For example, human ESC may differentiate spontaneously and yield an undesirable product.

To understand the complexity of research into stem cells—human embryonic stem cells in particular—refer to Table 4.1. ESC as a therapy presents problems similar to those of organ transplantation. It would be an option of last resort, and the recipient may live a few more years, all the while maintained on immunosuppressants. Three other procedures have been suggested as possibilities: therapeutic cloning, stem cell gene therapy, and directed differentiation of the patient's own stem cells.

Therapeutic cloning is the deliberate creation of an embryo using somatic transfer technology (cloning) to produce a compatible human

Table 4.1 Human Embryonic Stem Cells: Issues to Be Addressed

Situation	Questions to Answer
Source and control	What source controls must be put in place for donated stem cell tissue?
	Are existing standards for donated blood or organs good enough?
	Will there be complications from blood-borne pathogens, especially when stem cells are used as a basis for cell lines?
	If cells are used for cell lines, should donors be required to undergo additional tests?
Record keeping	What records need to be kept of the end use of donated tissue?
	How long would such records need to be kept, and who should have access to them?
	If detailed history notes are not kept, could they still be considered safe for use?
Safety issues	Should genetic testing be done prior to use of donated testing in cell lines?
	Which tests should be done? Are the existing tests sufficiently sensitive and reliable?
	What happens when hESCs or hEGCs prove positive for neurodegenerative disease?
	Are some types of stem cells inherently safer than others?
Purity	Do isolation and maintenance procedures used distinguish between desirable and undesirable cell lines?
	Will purity of any final product be assured? If not, what level of impurity, in the form of heterogeneous mixture, would be acceptable?
	Are there markers that will verify accurately that the correct cell types have been produced? Are there markers that can be used to eliminate cell types that may be inherently dangerous?
Potency	How will potency be defined?

Source: Developed by Evelyn B. Kelly.

embryonic stem cell line. In the process, a skin cell is taken from the patient and injected into eggs from which the nucleus has been removed. When the embryo reaches the blastocyst stage, the scientist isolates and cultures the inner cell mass. Then growth factors or other procedures stimulate the required tissue differentiation. Because the tissue is the patient's own, there will be no antigens to cause rejection. The process is still theoretical and will be very expensive to carry out. In addition, ethical baggage attaches.

Stem cell gene therapy is the process of harvesting stem cells from patients with genetic diseases. In an **ex vivo** (out of the body) process, DNA—usually composed of the entire coding region of a gene along with its regulatory sequences—is added to the cells containing the defective gene. The area of the specific defect is targeted, and the gene is added for correction. This is called genetic editing. The corrected gene is then put back into the body using a vector. Another gene therapy process uses an engineered stock culture to carry cell-surface antigens that would be acceptable to the patient's immune system. In theory it would be much better to engineer the patient's own stem cells, but this would be an even more expensive process than therapeutic cloning.

Directed differentiation could occur in adult stem cells. Although embryonic cells exhibit more plasticity, scientists are excited about the regenerative-medicine possibilities in adult stem cells. The patient's own stem cells can be used for the process of differentiation. A routine bone marrow tap can yield adult stem cells that can be cultured and then coaxed to differentiate into the needed tissue. Catherine Verfallie, a University of Minnesota researcher, challenged the prevailing theory that adult stem cells are not plastic when she and colleagues found that certain stem cells isolated from adult bone marrow may have the same plasticity as human embryonic stem cells. Another Minnesota colleague, Juliet Barker, found that stem cells from the umbilical cord also demonstrate a high degree of plasticity. This research has really expanded in the last few years and, with the additional development of the right growth factors, growth of tissues from adult stem cells will explode in the near future.

New procedures for harvesting stem cells—adult stem cells in particular— appear often in the literature. Jeffrey Bourley (2005) discovered and reported on a procedure developed at the University of Cincinnati that shows how blood-regenerating stem cells move from the bone marrow into the bloodstream. This led to the development of a new chemical compound that can accelerate the process of stem cell mobilization in mice. This procedure could eventually lead to more efficient stem cell harvesting for human use and potential therapeutics. Bourley's findings appeared in the

August 6, 2005, issue of *Nature Medicine* and are interesting because they involve harvesting adult stem cells, not embryonic stem cells.

Cincinnati scientists Jose Cancelas and David Williams (2005) found that a family of proteins called RAC GTPase play a significant role in regulating the movement of stem cells into the bone marrow. By inhibiting this protein, they were able to instruct stem cells to move from the bone marrow and into the bloodstream, where they can be more easily collected. However, moving from the mouse model to the human model could prove time-consuming, and there currently are no target dates for development.

Stem cells have been found in unexpected places. David Cyranoski and Declan Butler (2006) reported on the work of Gerd Hasenfuss and colleagues from the University of Gottingen, Sweden. The researchers found a potential source of reprogrammable cells taken from the testes. They extracted the cells from male mice, but speculated that it should be possible to produce similar results from human testicles through biopsy. To perform the work, the team created a transgenic breed of mice in which sperm-producing stem cells were labeled with a fluorescent marker. They then cultured the stem cells using typical materials and found that some of them looked like embryonic cells. They then tagged these cells with a blue marker and injected them into young mouse embryos to see whether they had the power to develop inside a living mouse. In 90 percent of the cases, they did.

PROCEDURE FOR HUMAN TRIALS

The procedure to advance to human testing is complex and time-consuming. It may follow steps such as these:

- Human embryonic stem cells are used to establish pure cultures of specific cell types.
- Investigators test the physiologic function. For example, in vitro the scientist may test for a specific stimulated response, such as how insulin reacts.
- Investigators demonstrate efficacy first in rodents and then in nonhuman primates. They also demonstrate safety in nonhuman primates, ensuring the absence of tumor formation and infectious agents, and taking care that the cells not be rejected.
- Human trials will slowly develop.

This chapter has considered some practical problems with the growing and testing of stem cells. Chapters 5, 6, and 7 will look at specific systems and at diseases and disorders related to stem cell research.

CHAPTER 5

Hope for the Future: Diseases and Disorders of the Nervous System

On 16 July 2005, tiny Timea Gresco was born three months early in a small town in Hungary. When she began to have tremors, it was evident that something was wrong. Timea could move her limbs only at a reduced rate, like slow motion, and her left side had less movement than the right. She cried incessantly, never smiled, and did not acknowledge anyone's presence. The doctors said that she was probably the youngest person ever to suffer a stroke.

Timea's mother, Judit Godo, had heard of a procedure developed by the Chinese biotechnology company Shenzhen Beike. Due to Hungarian regulations, this procedure could not be performed on Timea in her own country; Timea and her mother traveled to China. For two months, umbilical cord stem cells were fed into her tiny veins.

Now Timea is a much improved baby. She smiles a lot and eats her food—something she would not do previously. Her left arm is just about as strong as her right, and she no longer keeps her head to one side. Timea will go back to China for another treatment when she turns one year old, but right now, her condition looks positive. Currently, procedures like the one used to treat Timea—using umbilical cord blood to treat neurological diseases—are not performed in the United States because of the amount of time required to secure Food and Drug Administration (FDA) approval. China is leading in the investigation of cord blood research.

Stem cell research has advanced our knowledge of how organisms develop as well as of how healthy cells can replace damaged cells in an adult. In this promising area, scientists are investigating the possibility of cell-based therapies to treat disease. Often referred to as regenerative or reparative medicine, this area of biology is one of today's most promising. Questions are raised with each new discovery, and many challenges must be conquered before the dream of regenerative medicine becomes a reality. This chapter, and Chapters 6 and 7, lay the foundation for work in many areas. This chapter considers the possibilities for treatment of the brain and spinal cord.

RESEARCH INTO THE NERVOUS SYSTEM

At one time, it was thought that brain cells did not grow and reproduce. It was assumed that a person was born with a certain number of cells and this did not change; destruction of the cells meant that the brain would deteriorate. Research into the brain in the past few decades has changed that paradigm. Scientists now believe that the adult central nervous system (CNS) may have the capacity for regeneration and repair. This greatly expands the possibilities for future treatment of CNS disorders, offering potential strategies for treating the entire scope of neurological diseases.

Ample evidence exists that stem cells remain in the CNS throughout life, and that these cells may have the ability to assume the functional role of neural cells that have been lost. The CNS is a prime target for embryonic stem cell therapy. There is no doubt that stem cells can survive, migrate, and differentiate. Stem cells offer hope for several disorders, such as Alzheimer's disease (AD), Parkinson's disease (PD), Tay-Sachs disease, Huntington's disease, spinal cord trauma, and stroke. However, progress on the nervous system is difficult because of a complex of different kinds of cells that make it difficult to focus on the system itself. See the sidebar Short Course on the Brain and Neurons. As of 2006, most researchers believe that stem cell therapies for nervous system disorders may not be available for 10 to 20 years.

Neural stem cells have been isolated from both the developing embryo and the adult brain. The driving force behind deciphering the developmental program is related to understanding cell fate, or what makes the cell differentiate. Fate decisions appear to be made in the ectoderm from the **neuroepithelial cells (NECs)** of the **neural plate.** The term **neural induction** refers to the early events that lead to the formation of the NEC of the neural tube, where the progenitor cells give rise to the neurons and glial cells. **Neural patterning** refers to the developmental processes in which the precursors are positioned to give rise to the subtype of neurons from a complex network of gene expression.

ALZHEIMER'S DISEASE

In 1907 Dr. Alois Alzheimer, a German physician, described a patient whose bizarre behavior was accompanied by progressive memory and language loss as well as the increasing inability to recognize friends. When the patient died, he studied slides of her brain and found that they were a tangled mass of threads of dead neurons and plaque-like deposits. The condition that now bears his name, Alzheimer's disease, is a devastating neurological disorder affecting 5.5 million adults in the United States.

AD begins in the **hippocampus,** an area of the brain important for coordinating memory functions. During the early stages of AD, an individual may exhibit some change in personality but not enough to raise concerns. As years pass, the tangles and plaques spread to other parts of the cerebrum and the person appears confused and forgetful. Three genes have been implicated for the cause of AD: *tau,* which codes for a needed protein, *App* (amyloid precursor protein), and *Sen,* or presenilin, which codes for needed enzymes. Defects in any or all of these genes can lead to the neural death that is characteristic of AD.

Stem cells have been stimulated to differentiate into neurons and glial cells. Experiments with mouse models of AD have shown that stem cells that have been injected directly into the brain can produce functional neurons near the plaque lesions. Scientists do not know yet if these neurons will make the correct connection and be able to replace the complex damage caused by AD.

PARKINSON'S DISEASE

In 1817 Dr. James Parkinson, an English physician, described a condition in which people, usually over the age of 50, slowly lose their motor control. The condition has specific symptoms. Generally, the person's hands begin to shake, the face will take on a frozen, mask-like expression, and the limbs become stiff and rigid. The mask-like facial expression may become fixed, with eyes that do not blink, and a mouth that may remain open with drooling saliva. The person will have difficulty walking; the posture becomes stooped and the gait may take the form of small baby steps, a movement sometimes called "march of the little feet." The person will also have difficulty maintaining his or her balance as the limbs become increasingly stiff and rigid. Scientists now know that this condition affects neurons in an area of the midbrain called the substantia nigra, which controls motor coordination. Progressive degeneration and loss of the dopamine-producing neurons cause Parkinson's disease. The degeneration leads to the tremors, rigidity, and abnormally reduced mobility called hypokinesia. Scientists surmise that Parkinson's is inherited, and strongly suspect a gene on chromosome 4.

At the onset of clinical symptoms, the majority of dopamine-producing neurons have already died, making a good case for treatment by cell replacement. Several other factors support this rationale:

- Neurological damage is restricted to one area of the brain.
- A specific cell type, the dopamine-producing neurons, is needed to relieve the symptoms of this disease.
- Preclinical animal research has shown that stem cells can be stimulated into becoming neurons that produce the neurotransmitter dopamine.
- Injection of neuronal stem cells into the brains of Parkinson mouse models has relieved some of the motor deficits in the mouse.

Several laboratories have been successful in developing embryonic cells that, after differentiation, can perform many of the functions of dopamine-producing neurons. Scientists have found an animal model of PD. A recent study found that mouse embryonic stem cells differentiate into dopamine-producing neurons by introducing the gene Nurr1. When transplanted into the rat model, these cells cause healthy new cells to grow.

Transplantation of stem cells in the model has shown that a large number of cells can grow in the midbrain; however, a downside is that teratomas develop. Several issues must be resolved before clinical trials with human embryonic stem cell (hES)-derived dopamine can come about. Twenty years of fetal research have shown that fetal midbrain dopamine can live more than ten years, but with limited efficacy and potential side effects. To move to the next level, fetal transplantation trials must address critical parameters. Finding highly purified populations of substantia nigra dopamine neurons for hES is an important first step on this road.

PD is a common neurodegenerative disorder affecting more than 2 percent of the population over 65 years of age—4.5 million people. It is one of the most widely discussed applications for stem cell transplantation, and patients with PD may be the first to receive a stem cell–based treatment.

HUNTINGTON'S DISEASE (HD)

In 1872 Dr. George Huntington documented a condition in which victims in their early thirties developed quick, jerky, involuntary movements, double vision, and slow mental degeneration. Named after Dr. Huntington, this condition is sometimes called the "Crown Jewel of Research" because the gene that causes it has been located on a specific chromosome. HD is similar to Parkinson's disease in that it affects a specific and selective neuronal population: the GABAergic medium spiny neurons in an area of the midbrain called the **striatum.** Fetal transplantation experiments have supported the concept of cell-based treatments of the disease. It is unlike PD in that the cells do not connect to local cells within the striatum but must project to targets in the area of the brain adjacent to the substantia nigra. Embryonic stem cell–derived GABAergic neurons have not been tested yet in any animal model of HD, but in vitro experiments with GABAergic neurons showed efficiency. Another possible avenue for stem cells in the treatment of HD is the derivation of stem cells from embryos with HD mutations.

SPINAL CORD AND OTHER INJURIES

When a person is in a serious impact accident or falls from a high place, damage to the spinal cord can keep the brain from controlling the body's extremities and organs. Christopher Reeve, the actor famous for portraying Superman, was thrown from a horse and broke his neck. A quadriplegic after the accident, Reeve was unable to move his arms or legs and could not breathe properly. He became a strong proponent of stem cell research.

If the damage occurs lower on the back, the person may retain control of the arms and lungs but be able to use the legs. Injury to the spinal cord damages the neurons that lead to specific parts of the body, and is devastating and usually irreversible.

Victims of spinal cord injuries have received much publicity for their support of stem cell research, but hope is probably the only thing they have at present. Cell replacement in this area is complex and difficult to resolve for several reasons:

- Damaged neurons must be replaced before the function can be restored.
- The replacement neurons must make the proper connections to the damaged area.
- Once the neurons are replaced, the myelin sheath must insulate them just as they are insulated in the normal body. See the sidebar Short Course on the Brain and Neurons.

Motor neurons lead the brain's electrical impulses to the muscles and organs. They are involved in both spinal injuries and conditions like amyotrophic lateral sclerosis (ALS), or Lou Gehrig's disease. Scientists have derived motor neurons from ESC and injected them into a developing chick's spinal cord with some success. Dr. Ronald McKay, a researcher at the National Institutes of Health, has shown that mouse ESC can repair some neural damage in rats. The behavior of these cells when injected into humans is yet to be tested.

In November 2005 Dr. Brian Cummins from the University of California at Irvine found that human neural stem cells can replace damaged cells and improve function in a mouse model of spinal cord injury. The team injected the cells into the site of the injury and followed the progress. The cells survived, grafted with the injured mouse spinal cord, and persisted 17 weeks after transplantation. The injected stem cells formed neurons and synapses, and the mice showed evidence of recovering coordinated motor function and stepping ability 16 weeks after the grafts. According to the researchers, there is hope; it is just a long way off. The study was conducted with very controlled injuries and resulted only in improved function. The mice were not cured. Cummings observed that future treatments will require a combination of therapies because spinal injuries are very complex and no single treatment will solve the problem.

STROKE

A stroke might be called a brain attack. A blockage of blood flow or bleeding (hemorrhage) in the brain causes a stroke. The person may experience sudden numbness or paralysis of the face, arm, or leg. Other common signs include loss of speech, blurred vision, dizziness, or sudden headaches. The medical term for stroke is cerebrovascular event or disease, which indicates that it originates in the blood vessels of the brain. Location and type of disturbance characterize a stroke. A common type is called **ischemia,** when the blood supply through an artery is deficient. When this happens, tissues and cells that depend on that blood die quickly. Time is very important in warding off damage.

Transplantation of stem cells is complicated because there are so many different locations and types of cell populations. According to Lorenz Studer (2006), a recent study showed that grafted ESC can survive in a rat stroke model. He found extensive migration of the grafted cells along the corpus collosum toward the lesion caused by the stroke. Other than this one experiment, little information is available about the behavior of ESC in animal models of stroke.

DISEASES THAT CAUSE DEMYELINATION

The myelin sheath provides insulation and protection for the neurons, which do not function properly when this covering is damaged, causing the person to experience numbness, tingling, tremors, impaired gait, or other motor problems. One of the major conditions of the myelin sheaths is multiple sclerosis (MS), a disease that comes and goes and is the chief cause of disability among adults of working age. The condition may start between the ages of 20 and 40.

Mouse models of MS have been shown to respond to ESC-derived glial cells where large numbers of **oligodendrocytes** were grown. Multiple sclerosis is particularly problematic because of its autoimmune nature. An autoimmune condition is one in which the body's own immune system thinks the cells are outside enemies, and attacks them. Many conditions, including arthritis and scleroderma, are autoimmune diseases.

AMYOTROPHIC LATERAL SCLEROSIS (ALS), OR LOU GEHRIG'S DISEASE

Lou Gehrig was a baseball player for the New York Yankees during the Babe Ruth glory years. He was a favorite of the fans and was pleasant and humble. After several years, coaches and fans noted that Gehrig was struggling in his game; eventually he revealed he had a disease that would be fatal. The disease caused him to gradually lose control of movement. The condition, amyotrophic lateral sclerosis (ALS), is commonly called "Lou Gehrig's disease" after this famous player.

ALS is a progressive disease. Its gradual evolution includes a general spreading weakness and wasting of the affected patient's muscles. It leads to dysfunction, disability, chronic ventilator dependency, and death—usually three years after weakness is first detected. The direct cause of muscle weakness and wasting is the progressive loss of the muscle's motor neurons. The affected motor nerve cells reside in the spinal cord where nerves are connected to muscles directly. Upper motor neurons—nerve cells and circuits involved in higher-order planning, thinking, and sequencing—reside in the anterior portion of the brain, and also may be affected.

No treatment exists that can halt or reverse the course of ALS. The FDA has approved riluzole as a treatment, but this may add only two or three months to patients' mean survival, which certainly is not acceptable. Stem cells could help ALS patients in several ways:

- Stem cells could be induced to differentiate into lower motor neurons to replace those neurons that die because of ALS.
- Stem cells could rescue dying motor neurons by connecting these neurons to a partly denervated muscle before it has died completely.

- Stem cells could be induced to differentiate into upper motor neurons in the cortex that connect to the lower motor neurons.
- Stem cells might be induced into becoming supporting cells for glia, or becoming interneurons that might produce factors that could support motor neurons.

All of these tasks are very complex and fairly unrealistic. The last possibility might be the most feasible. A. M. Clement and colleagues (2003) studied genetically engineered mice whose motor neurons carried an abnormal SOD1 gene (a gene found in families with ALS) and whose glial, or supportive, cells carried a healthy gene. The scientists found that survival times in those mice were extended compared with mice that had abnormal genes in both the motor and glial cells. This suggests that if healthy stem cells could get to the spinal cords of patients with ALS, their survival might be extended.

The ethics of performing human studies at this early stage of stem cell research has been questioned because of the risks of premature human trials. Reports of stem cell transplantation performed in China without peer review of objective data do not provide sufficient scientific evidence to demonstrate that the treatment is safe and effective.

THE EYE AND EAR

Human beings rely heavily on the senses of sight and hearing. It is unfortunate that both deteriorate with age. Diseases that affect the eyes and ears are difficult to treat, and few therapies are available. Thus, as stem cell research has promised hope for patients suffering from other diseases, stem cell research designed to benefit eyes and ears has also accelerated.

The eye has an opening at the front called the pupil, which lets in light. The light is regulated by the opening and closing of the colored part of the eye, the iris. On the back of the eye is the retina, which completely lines the inner surface of the eye and is made of an abundance of different kinds of specialized sensory receptor cells called rods and cones. The nerve cells and nerve processes responsible for vision are found within the retina. Nerve fibers on the receptor rods and cones all pass across the innermost surface of the retina and unite at the back of the eye to form the optic nerve.

The retina is a model of central nervous system anatomy, physiology, and development. Finding retinal stem cells has been the goal of recent studies. Retinal neurons and glia from retinal progenitor cells are considered to be multipotent. One approach to finding stem cells has been to search for mitotic cells capable of generating retinal neurons in the adult in vivo. The other approach has been to culture cells using growth factors. Both procedures may be promising.

The eye originates from the neural tube, the neural crest, the surface ectoderm, and the mesoderm during embryonic development. A structure called the optic cup forms the retina, and the outer part of the cup develops a nonneural structure—the retinal pigmented epithelium, or RPE—to capture stray light that passes through the retina. Both the inner and outer parts of the cup form the iris and the ciliary body that control the contraction and expansion of the iris. Stem cells have been isolated from the ciliary body, the iris, and the glia of the retina in young chicks.

A large number of diseases of the retina are caused by degeneration of the rod cells. In fact, about 40 percent of the genes identified for blindness are specific to the rods, structures that are sensitive to low levels of white light. However, the death of the cones is responsible for the loss of high-acuity daylight vision. Macular degeneration, in which the individual loses central vision, is of special interest although the exact cause is unknown.

The ear is composed of three areas: (1) the external ear, which includes the ear canal; (2) the middle ear, or tympanic cavity, which includes the three bones of the ossicles and the eardrum; and (3) the inner ear. The inner ear is the most important part of the auditory apparatus because it contains the cochlea, a structure that resembles a small snail shell with a spiral canal that houses tiny hair-like projections called cilia. These cilia receive sound vibrations and translate them into nerve impulses that proceed down the auditory nerve to a special area in the brain.

The entire structure of the ear develops from the ectoderm. Several groups of scientists have used **oncogenes,** a mutant form of a normal cellular gene, to isolate cell lines from the developing ear and explore their differentiation potential. Methods for culturing **otic** stem cells are being developed. When the cells are differentiated, they may then be transplanted back into the animal model to investigate whether cells will integrate and restore the auditory function. The ear may have some advantages because it is particularly well suited to gene therapy delivery vectors such as viruses and surgery. Technical progress is expected in ear therapy over the next decade, although several hurdles exist.

Scientists have come a long way in understanding how the brain works and operates. However, the complexity of brain structures and the types of neurons and supporting cells make therapeutic work very difficult. Unfortunately, it will probably be 10 to 20 years before we see breakthroughs in treating the nervous system diseases and disorders.

A Short Course on the Brain and Neurons

Neurons, or Nerve Cells

Although neurons vary in size and shape, they have three basic parts: axon, cell body, and dendrite. Electrical impulses flowing in one direction enter the neuron through the branched dendrite, move through the cell body, exit through the axon, and then go across the synapse (or gap) to the dendrite of the next neuron. Chemical neurotransmitters, such as dopamine and serotonin, assist the movement of the impulse across the synapse. Axons are insulated with a sheath of shiny, white material called myelin that protects and insulates. Myelin is made from oligodendrocytes and **Schwann cells.** There are three types of neurons:
- Sensory neurons, which receive impulses from the sense organs
- Motor neurons, which carry impulses to muscles
- Associative neurons, which relay impulses from sensory to motor neurons and are located in the brain and spinal cord

Brain

The brain is made of three parts: cerebrum, cerebellum, and brain stem.
- The cerebrum is the thinking part of the brain. Its main portion, the cerebral cortex, is home to our intellect and personality, and analyzes sensory information. Located deep in the brain, the hippocampus coordinates memory function.
- The cerebellum controls coordination and movement.
- The brain stem controls many of our automatic processes, like breathing and the beating of the heart. Near the top of the brain stem is the substantia nigra, which contributes to balance and walking. The brain stem is made of three parts: the pons, the midbrain, and the medulla oblongata, which connects to the spinal cord.

The halves of the brain are connected by a tough, band-like material called the corpus collosum. Brain scientists have located many subdivisions of each of the parts of the brain.

CHAPTER 6

Of Blood, Bones, and the Immune System

On May 18, 2005, a 61-year-old man entered Saitama Medical Center in Kanwagoe, Japan, with severe chest pains and all the symptoms of a heart attack. Earlier, in February, he had received an external artificial heart. Because of his age and other factors, the patient was judged unsuitable for a heart transplant, but Dr. Shunel Kyo and assistants were ready to attempt a new feat. They took stem cells from the patient's bone marrow and injected them into the man's heart. On June 30, the patient was doing so well, the artificial heart was removed. Doctors were pleased with the patient's progress and saw this trial as a possible breakthrough. However, they recognized that further scientific data would have to be collected; the one success was not enough on which to make snap decisions about new uses for stem cells.

Moving stem cells from basic and applied research in animals to clinical practice is the goal of regenerative medicine. Cases such as the one from Japan (and other parts of the world) are encouraging but by no means conclusive. One of the most promising possibilities for the use of stem cells is in treating conditions of the blood and heart.

MAKING BLOOD CELLS

British poet and essayist Alice Meynell wrote, "The true color of life is the color red of the living heart and the pulses." Most people think very little about how the circulating red blood beneath the skin transports oxygen, nourishment, and disease-fighting substances. Only if there is a blood disease or a problem with the heart do we begin to appreciate the life-giving flow.

After the brain, the most important tissue of the human body is blood. Blood tissue accounts for about 8 percent of total body weight, and is made of several components:

- *Plasma.* Plasma constitutes about 55 percent of the blood. It is a brownish, watery liquid containing dissolved substances, mostly proteins.
- *Red blood cells (RBCs), or erythrocytes.* These oxygen transporters contain a protein called hemoglobin. They number about 4.8 to 5.4 million per cubic millimeter.
- *White blood cells, or leukocytes.* These immune system cells number about 5,000 to 10,000 per cubic millimeter.
- *Platelets or thrombocytes.* These cell fragments are involved in blood clotting and number about 250,000 to 400,000 per cubic millimeter.

The three blood cells—erythrocytes, leukocytes, and thrombocytes—make up about 45 percent of the blood and are carried in the plasma.

Blood cells are formed in a process called hematopoiesis. During embryonic and fetal development, the following centers are important for producing blood cells: the yolk sac, liver, spleen, thymus gland, lymph nodes, and bone marrow. After birth, hematopoiesis occurs mostly in the red bone marrow, or myeloid tissue, found in the upper end of the long bones of the arm (humerus) and thigh (femur), in flat bones such as the sternum and cranial bones, and in the vertebrae and pelvic bones.

The cells that give rise to differentiated blood cells are called hematoblasts. These pluripotent hematopoietic cells differentiate into the several types of blood cells. The home of most hematoblasts is the red bone marrow, although some primary cells may circulate in the blood. From these primary precursors come secondary precursor cells: erythroblasts, myeloblasts, monoblasts, lymphoblasts, and megakaryoblasts.

The mad rush to discover the source of human blood began in the second half of the nineteenth century when Paul Ehrlich (1854–1915) developed techniques for staining microscopic slides of blood with aniline dyes that enabled him to categorize blood cells. German pathologist Carl Heitzmann (1836–1896) had published an earlier paper announcing he had discovered the primary blood cells, which he called hematoblasts—from the Greek *hemo,* meaning "blood," and *blast,* meaning "give birth to." Georges Hayem, a French scientist who is sometimes called the father of hematology, refined the staining of the blood cells and published a popular textbook on diseases of the blood in 1887.

In 1961, James Till and Ernest McCullough identified the hematopoietic stem cell. They noted the cell's ability to self-renew in the marrow and differentiate into the full complement of cell types found in adult stem cells. Hematopoietic stem cells are among the few to be isolated in adult humans. Scientists found that they normally reside in the bone marrow but under some conditions migrate to other tissues through the blood. They are also normally found in the fetal liver and spleen, and in umbilical and placental blood.

In 2001 Orlic et al. found that injection of bone marrow into injured hearts promotes restoration of function. Using antibody staining, the researchers traced donor cells that expressed myocardial markers. They surmised that stem cells were able to differentiate into the myocardium and replace injured tissue. Other researchers did not replicate this finding, but the discussion encouraged others to begin to investigate the new technique of cell fusion. In this procedure, cells from a donor fuse with cells of an independent lineage.The fused cell often expresses the differentiation markers of the host cell but also carries markers of both cells.

THE HEART

The heart is the first of the organs to develop in the embryo. A healthy heart will continue to work from the very first beat throughout a lifetime— on average, a total of more than 2.5 billion beats.

Researchers have used stem cells from a variety of sources to attack the problems of the heart. Sources include bone marrow–derived stem cells, peripheral blood-derived stem cells, embryonic stem cells, umbilical cord blood cells, and muscle-derived cells.

Bone Marrow–Derived Stem Cells

Bone marrow appears to have three stem cell populations: hematopoietic, endothelial progenitor, and mesenchymal cells (mSCs) that have the potential for multiple lineages of differentiation. The stem cells from the marrow are responsible for the renewal of blood cells and exhibit constant self-renewal. Mesenchymal stem cells are mixed populations that generate bone, cartilage, fat, connective tissue, and the network that supports blood cell formation. However, testing in bovine models has shown that undifferentiated hSCs will become functional cardiac muscle, able to avoid destruction by the host immune system.

M. Kudo et al. (2003) injected two types of bone marrow–derived stem cells into the injured myocardium (i.e., the heart muscle) and extracted **Lin cells** (an enriched type of mSC) and cultured mSCs. The Lin cells engrafted in the damaged area, differentiated into cardiomyocytes and vascular cells, and reduced the size and scarring of the **infarct** (i.e., the damaged area). Other groups have shown that autologous cells from the patient's own bone marrow are beneficial in improving heart function in animals and humans.

This research into transplants has shown that **cardiomyocytes** (i.e., cells of the heart muscle) can form a connection—a functional **syncytium**—with the host myocardium. Muscle cells from the heart are attractive because they can be obtained from animal and human sources. Cell transplantation has emerged as a potential therapeutic intervention to restore muscle lost in diseased hearts. However, there are some limitations: (1) no markers exist to identify lost heart muscle, and (2) the most effective method of delivering the cell to the heart has not been established.

However, the full potential of bone marrow transplantation to restore a healthy heart and blood system is currently limited by the quantity and purity of hSCs. They are relatively rare, occurring at a rate of only one in 10,000 bone marrow cells. Because of the difficulty of separating hSCs from other cells, they are relatively impure. This impurity is very important because the host body may reject cells as foreign, and may cause the T-cells to attack the implant. This lethal condition is known as graft-versus-host disease (GVHD). Autologous implantation may solve the problem, but may create another one—the problem of bringing into the implant diseased or cancerous cells. Transplants from cord blood and placenta usually are easier to purify but are difficult to obtain in large amounts.

Peripheral Blood–Derived Stem Cells

Cells isolated from adult human peripheral blood have been shown to differentiate into various tissues. One study found that **CD34+ cells** isolated from blood and injected into the tail vein in mice were able to move to the infarct zone and differentiate into cardiomyocytes, endothelial cells, and smooth muscle cells. In this experiment, administration of ascorbic acid helped the types to differentiate.

K. Ogawa et al. (2004) injected these blood cells into a patient with an enlarged heart. The patient improved but lost the benefit of cell therapy after ten months. This experiment showed that peripheral blood cells may be of clinical value in the future, but the time frame and effective cell numbers warrant further investigation.

Embryonic Stem Cells

It has been established that embryonic cells can differentiate into functional heart cells in vitro and that these cell-derived cardiomyocytes could be suitable for implantation. The efficacy of ESC-derived transplantation has been validated in experimental animals.

Umbilical Cord Blood Cells

Stem cells from umbilical cord have been shown to be rich in progenitor cells that can proliferate. One scientist showed that infused CD133+ cells derived from human umbilical cord can migrate, colonize, and survive in the myocardium of infarcted rats. Some of the cells in the damaged area were able to form new heart tissue. The cells also prevented scarring and dysfunction of the left ventricle. Work in this area is still in its infancy, but results thus far indicate cord blood cells' strong potential to repair damaged heart tissue.

On March 1, 2006, the Cooper Heart Institute in Camden, New Jersey, partnered with the Coriell Institute for Medical Research in a study examining the role of stem cells in repairing damaged hearts. The Cooper Institute's Dr. Joseph Parrillo believes these studies represent the first step in a path that promises to treat—and potentially to cure—heart disease without transplantation or other complex surgery. Dr. Steven Hollenberg, director of Cooper's coronary care unit, considers cord blood to be the holy grail of stem cell research in cardiology. Treatment with cord blood cells has been shown to make new heart muscle and to make cells that help the heart pump more efficiently.

Seeding donor cells in numbers sufficient to directly affect cardiac function and donor cell rejection are hurdles to be overcome. Once they are, cellular transplantation will arise as a promising treatment for heart disease.

Muscle-Derived Cells

Skeletal muscle is able to regenerate and repair itself when injured. It is an interesting property of these cells that they are capable of fusing with other myoblasts or surrounding cells to produce functional skeletal muscle. Myoblasts represent an exciting possibility in cell therapy research: they can be easily obtained from a muscle biopsy, grown in culture, and then readily returned without risk of immunosuppression and without the ethical problems that arise when researchers work with embryonic cells.

LEUKEMIA

Each year in the United States, nearly 32,000 adults and more than 2,000 children develop leukemia, a cancer of the blood. Leukemia affects only white blood cells and has two forms: (1) acute, which quickly destroys the patient's immune system; and (2) chronic, which progresses more slowly. Standard treatment for leukemia now involves radiation and chemotherapy that may completely destroy the bone marrow and require bone marrow transplantation. If an acceptable donor is not available, the patient's outlook is not good.

Stem cells isolated from the marrow of the affected patient can be induced to differentiate into normal white blood cells and then be grown in culture to increase in number. The stem cells are then returned to the patient to reconstitute as healthy, cancer-free bone marrow.

On December 20, 2005, Osiris Therapeutics in Baltimore, Maryland, announced that it had received orphan drug designation from the U.S. Food and Drug Administration (FDA) for its adult stem cell product, Prochymal, under investigation for use in the treatment of acute graft-versus-host disease (GVHD). This formulation has the ability to modulate the immune system in a way that may benefit patients suffering from a variety of immunological disorders. Two studies are taking place for the treatment of GVHV, a complication of bone marrow transplantation. GVHD is a life-threatening immune disorder that affects about 50 percent of patients who receive donated bone marrow transplants for treatment of cancers such as leukemia.

IMMUNE DEFICIENCIES

The immune system is designed to battle invaders. Without it, living beings would face death from overwhelming infection. The immune system is a complex of white blood cells that appear in several forms:

- Granulocytes—made of neutrophils, basophils, and eosinophils that have a distinct granular nucleus and are phagocytic (i.e., able to eat cells, viruses, and debris).
- Monocytes—large cells that are phagocytic and have one nucleus. Macrophages, the largest member of the monoctye group, can engulf entire bacteria and damaged or aging cells. They are the body's first line of defense.
- Lymphocytes—smooth and round and having a large, round nucleus. Three main types of lymphocytes are (1) **B lymphocytes,** which are nonphagocytic but able to produce antibodies; (2) **T lymphocytes,** sometimes known as killer T-cells; and (3) **natural killer (NK) cells.** T cells and NK cells direct the immune response.

SEVERE COMBINED IMMUNODEFICIENCY (SCID)

Many conditions affect the immune system. Severe combined immuno-deficiency-X1 (SCID) is a rare disease that destroys the immune response. This condition is inherited and usually carried on the X chromosome. Males receive this sex-linked gene from a carrier mother and die within the first few years of life. Photographs of David, the smiling "Bubble

Boy" who lived his 12-year life completely enclosed in a sterile plastic bag, drew attention to this disease.

A second form of SCID is a mutation in the adenosine deaminase (ADA) gene, located on chromosome 20. The gene is related to T lymphocytes of the immune system, and ADA is required for proper functioning of that system. If the gene is not functioning properly, adenosine toxins can build up in the cell, affecting the activity of the immune system. Gene therapy has been used to deliver to patients hematopoietic cells with a healthy copy of the gene. This process has been one of the most successful gene therapy experiments.

BLOOD DISEASES

Thalassemia, the world's most common inherited single-gene disorder, affects a person's ability to produce hemoglobin, the red blood cell protein that carries oxygen and nutrients to the cells. Using bone marrow transplants, physicians at Children's Hospital and Research Center in Oakland, California, have initiated the first cure of alpha thalassemia major.

Like thalassemia, sickle cell disease is incredibly common, affecting more than 72,000 people in the United States. People with sickle cell anemia produce structurally abnormal hemoglobin, which forms polymers that distort red blood cells into sickle shapes. These rigid cells become trapped in the small blood vessels, causing severe pain, organ damage, and sometimes stroke. The current therapeutic approach is to destroy all sickle cell–producing blood cells and replace them with healthy cells. Wiping out a child's complete immune system is a serious and painful procedure. Doctors at Children's Hospital are experimenting with the technique of suppressing or partly disabling the child's immune system, instead of completely wiping it out. This approach allows time for the donor cells to begin to grow.

With funding from the National Heart, Lung, and Blood Institute, Children's Hospital has established the world's only not-for-profit cord blood donor program. Cord blood—the blood that remains in the umbilical cord and placenta following birth—is a rich source of stem cells. Compared to bone marrow collection, the collection of cord blood is noninvasive, painless, less expensive, and relatively simple. If a family has a child with a transplantable condition, and a new brother or sister is expected, they may enroll in the Sibling Donor Cord Blood Program. This program processes blood from siblings with leukemia, cancer, or other transplantable illnesses. By the end of 2003, this donor program had released 43 units of cord blood, and 41 patients had received transplants. The world's first cord blood transplant was performed in 1988. Since then, more than 2,000 transplants have been performed.

Stem cell research involving heart and blood conditions is progressing well. The first successes of this science should soon be translating from basic research into clinical research.

CHAPTER 7

Tissue Engineering: Bones, Muscles, Skin, and Endocrine Glands

"My experience with multiple myeloma began in 1984 when I developed a very slow developing form of the bone cancer. In the fall of 2001 we decided that a stem cell transplant would be an option and reviewed the risks and side effects. We decided to do an autologous transplant, in which my own cells would be used."

"The first step was to take Cytoxan, a chemotherapy agent, to reduce my white blood cells. When the cell counts were very low, we were ready for the next phase—to collect enough peripheral stem cells that were free of cancer. Back in the hospital they gave me more chemo treatments to kill all my remaining white cells. Now I was left with no defenses at all to any communicable disease and had to stay in a special transplant ward. Receiving the stem cells was a great relief to me. Waiting to see if it was successful was agonizing, but after a week, doctors considered the levels high enough so that I could go home. While in the hospital I found painting and drawing were therapeutic. I had my MSU pillow, fun pajamas, and a singing moose that inhabited my IV pole."

"The transplant was successful, but I could not go out in public for 100 days, and I was in remission for about a year. Then the symptoms began to reemerge, and I have gone on to other treatment protocols."

Jim Niesen

Lapeer, Michigan

Jim Niesen's experience with stem cells is a story that we may not read about in the newspapers. Here is a person who endured the pain of chemotherapy and was full of hope as he received stem cells, only to have his symptoms begin to reoccur after a year. Jim expressed hope that the procedure would one day be effective. He died in March 2006. His experience shows that procedures that work in the laboratory may not always work with human patients.

The skeletal system is one of the first major targets for human research. Generally, the proof of principle has been shown in animal models. This chapter considers the progress of stem cell research in fighting diseases and disorders of the skeletal system and the endocrine system.

THE SKELETAL SYSTEM

From ancient times bones have fascinated people as an integral part of their ancient documents, literature, and art. Hebrew tradition tells how God caused a deep sleep to come over Adam and took out a rib to make woman. Adam recognized, "This is bone of my bone" (Genesis 1:28). Throughout history, bones have been associated with death and were thought to be dead. In fact, the word "skeleton" comes from the Greek word *skeletos,* meaning "dried up." However, people began to realize that this notion of bones being dead or dry was not true. Francois Rabelais (1484–1553), an irreverent French physician and author, wrote in *Gargantua and Panatgruel,* "Break the bones in two and suck up the life-giving marrow," perhaps one of the first documented suggestions that bones were alive and that the marrow had great value.

Embryologists and scientists today provide us with ample insight about bones and about the origins of the skeletal system in an individual. Around 12 days after conception, a band called the primitive streak appears along the back of the inner cell mass. This temporary structure will give rise to another temporary structure—the notocord—derived from the endoderm of the blastocyst and consisting of a rod of cells on the underside of the neural tube. On the side of the neural tube are tiny cube-like segments that will become the 31 spinal nerves that extend control to every part of the body. Around the middle of the fourth week, these cells differentiate into three groups:

- Cutis, which will develop into skin
- Muscle, situated on the inside of the cutis, which will become the muscles of the segment
- Sclerotome cells, which will form the core of the bone and cartilage

The vertebrate skeleton is composed of two specialized tissues—cartilage and bone—that surround and protect a third type of tissue, the bone marrow.

Each of the two skeletal tissues contains a specific cell type of mesenchymal origin: chondrocytes, which form cartilage, and **osteoblasts,** which form bone. Mesenchymal stem cells, also called marrow stromal cells, are adult stem cells found in the bone marrow that give rise to bone, fat, cartilage, and muscle cells. Both types of skeletal cells are critical for growth and maintenance of the skeleton. Chondrocytes are at the ends of bones and become the scaffolds of cartilage on which osteoblasts can deposit bone matrix during both prenatal and postnatal development. Osteoblasts synthesize a collagen-rich matrix that has the unique property of mineralization. A defect in any one of these two cells may cause one of a number of genetic and disease conditions.

Bone Fractures

According to Huang et al. (2006), more than 33 million musculoskeletal injuries occur in the United States each year. Bone appears to have the ability to regenerate itself with functional tissue that is similar to the original tissue; defects often heal spontaneously. However, cartilage, tendon, and ligament injuries usually result in replacement of the site by unorganized and inferior scar tissue.

Orthopedic work is still important. Bones may not heal properly, or a child may be born with congenital malformations in which bones require lengthening. Bone tumors or bone loss due to trauma are only a few of the myriad conditions that affect the skeletal system.

TISSUE ENGINEERING

In 1871 Theophilus Gluck cemented an ivory ball into a man's hip and started the search for making better bone. Later scientists harvested bone grafts from the person and other sources to replace worn and torn areas. Now, stem cell research is seeking not only to replace bone, but to generate new bone. The making of these tissues became known as tissue engineering.

When the term "tissue engineering" was introduced, it was based on the use of natural or synthetic scaffolds seeded with organ-specific cells ex vivo. In 1991, using marrow from a patient, Dr. John Connolly of the Orlando, Florida, Regional Medical Center concentrated the person's own cells using a centrifuge, a machine that separates substances using the whirling motion of centrifugal force. Connolly found that 18 of 20 tibial fractures treated with adult stem cells had healed. The adult stem cells, or pluripotent mesenchymal stem cells (mSCs), have the ability to differentiate into multiple mesodermal lineages and have been isolated from bone marrow, adipose (fat) tissue, and synovium. Here there appears to be an unlimited supply of cells that are easily harvested and can be expanded in tissue culture to large numbers. Another advantage is that these cells can be used in allogeneic transplants obtained from the patient's own cells.

Preclinical studies in a variety of animal models have demonstrated that bone marrow stromal cells, when used with appropriate carriers, can regenerate new bone. The wide variety of carriers range from collagen sponges to synthetic biodegradable polymers and hydroxyapatite derivatives.

The term **orthobiologics** is applied to biological solutions to orthopedic problems and the field of tissue engineering. Refining these procedures, George Mueschler and a team from Ohio's Cleveland Clinic took out stem cells, concentrated them, and grew them on a matrix. Tissue engineering today involves multiple and diverse disciplines using cells, materials, and bioactive factors in combination to restore and improve tissue function.

Tissue engineering's goal is developing techniques that will generate replacements for injured tissue. Three elements are required:

- Stem cells or other responsive cells
- Growth factors
- A scaffold, or matrix, to serve as a building block for cellular attachment, differentiation, and growing

Like the early embryo, the bone marrow harbors cells that go through the process of developing and form human mesenchymal stem cells. The second element, growth factors, is an important piece of the tissue engineering puzzle. University of California researcher Marshall Urist won a Nobel Prize in Physiology or Medicine for his work with proteins that control growth, called bone morphogenetic protein (BMP) and transforming growth factor (TGF). These factors revolutionized the field of orthopedics. The third piece, a scaffold, is something to build the bone on. Experimenters have used many materials, including calcium salts, ceramics, and coral. For example, George Mueschler and a team from Cleveland Clinic found that these cells could grow on a micro-patterned polymer that increases the growth of the cells by 280 percent. Futuristic plans involve using nanodevices to make a "smart scaffold" that would emit wireless signals with information on bone density and the progress of healing. This would assist the more than 500,000 patients who undergo bone grafts each year, and who dread the bone marrow transplant more than a root canal.

Stem cell–based tissue engineering represents a major turn in the concept of tissue engineering. The bioengineer must understand not only how cellular mechanisms work but also how structure relates to function—how well the graft will hold up under the stresses of every-day life. Consider, for example, the grueling torture that knees are exposed to just in simple living. Engineering of tendons and ligaments is still in its infancy; several scaffolds are in the experimental phase but are a long way from clinical trials.

Ligament and Tendons

These bands of dense connective tissues lend stability and provide movement for the joints. Injury to either of these can lead to significant decrease in function and to development of degenerative joint disease. The use of mSCs in gene therapy strategies has been successful in several animal models. Tissue engineering has combined stem cells with biodegradable scaffolds, enhancing the biomechanical properties of the normal tendon and ligaments.

Meniscus

According to Huang, the annual incidence of meniscal tears is approxi-mately 60 to 70 per 100,000. The menisci are semilunar cartilaginous structures that are essential for the working of the knee. Their main func-tion is load transmission during weight bearing, and they are important in shock absorption and joint lubrication. Surgical treatments now are not really effective.

Novel treatments in both growth factor–based and cell-based therapy options may be provided through mSCs. One possible strategy is prefabri-cation of a cartilage-like construct using stem cells and a biodegradable matrix. Data from rabbit studies have shown that mSCs embedded in a col-lagen sponge can enhance the formation of fibrocartilage at the defect site.

Osiris Therapeutics announced phase I and II clinical trials in 2005, to evaluate the safety and efficacy of its Chondrogen product for meniscal regeneration following partial surgery for damaged menisces. This study involved the adult stem cell mSC, which has shown benefit in animal models. The stem cells or placebo are injected one week after the surgery, and the recovery process is closely monitored by the orthopedic surgeon. The stem cells are from normal-health adult volunteer donors and are not derived from a fetus, embryo, or animal. Between 50 and 60 patients were recruited to participate in the trial.

Fat: A Stem Cell Goldmine

Every year in the United States some 567,810 liters of fat are removed for cosmetic or health purposes. This is tissue that may con-tain life-giving stem cells. Regenerative cells exist in high numbers in adipose tissues (body fat), one of the richest known sources of regenerative cells. Obviously, fat is a renewable resource—especially in the United States. These cells consist of adult stem cells, endothelial progenitor cells, and growth factor–producing cells. Fat is more easily removed than hematopoietic cells from bone marrow.

A handful of labs and biotechnology companies are exploring the use of adipose-derived stem cells (ASCs). One such lab is San Diego–based Macropore Biosurgery, which is working to extract stem cells for treatment in myocardial infarction. Other companies are researching treatments for Crohn's disease. Many questions remain about these cells and how therapeutically useful they may be.

TREATMENT OF DISEASES OF THE BONES

Two candidates for stem cell replacement are osteoporosis, a condition in which bone is lost after menopause, and osteogenesis imperfecta (OI), a genetic condition in which bone is brittle and breaks easily. OI is a defect of the type I collagen gene and is characterized by growth retardation, short stature, and numerous fractures because of fragile bones. Six children have enrolled in St. Jude Children's Research Hospital in Memphis, Tennessee, for intravenous administration of bone marrow from human leukocyte antigen (HLA) antigen-identical donors or from siblings. Five of the six patients showed engraftment in one or more sites, including bone, skin, and stroma. All showed an increase in growth during the six-month period afterward. Huang and colleagues attributed this increase to the generation of normal osteoblasts from the mSCs that were engrafted in the skeletal sites.

Osteoporosis

In osteoporosis, bones become porous and lose their density. The condition is associated with aging and hormonal changes primarily in women, although men also may experience the condition. The disease causes over 1.5 million fractures in the United States alone. The primary cause of the disease is that **osteoclasts** (cells that resorb bone) overcome the new bone that is formed by osteoblasts. Thus there is a progressive loss of bone, fracture, and deformity. Geron, a biotechnology company, has made osteoblasts from embryonic stem cells, which are now in preclinical trials in animals. If these trials are successful, plans are first to administer the cells to patients with fractures of the long bones of the leg or arm. Success here will lead to testing the cells on patients with severe osteoporosis.

AUTOIMMUNE DISEASES

With their rejuvenating properties, stem cells offer the potential for treatment or even cure of autoimmune and inflammatory diseases. Although the research is still in its infancy, scientists are looking for promising new therapeutic options for patients suffering from these conditions. Two autoimmune conditions that affect a large population are osteoarthritis (OA) and diabetes.

Osteoarthritis

Osteoarthritis is one of the oldest and most common conditions known to humankind. In the United States, this common degenerative joint disease affects an estimated 20.7 million adults (most over age 45) and may be responsible for more than 7 million physician visits per year. Originally, wear and tear on the joint was considered the main cause, but scientists now realize that inflammation plays a large role. In OA cartilage becomes thin, cracks, and breaks away, leaving the bone unprotected. Cartilage has poor healing ability, and superficial defects usually do not heal spontaneously. This is because the blood supply is poor, and the chondrocytes do not multiply readily. Patients have been treated with two techniques: (1) cartilage stimulation (drilling small holes in the cartilage) and (2) microfracture and replacement. These techniques never achieve restoration of the full function of native tissue, however.

Tissue engineering is a new development for cartilage defects. Cell-based therapy has already been used clinically with autologous chondrocytes. The cells are isolated from harvested cartilage and implanted for defects. Since 1987, more than 950 patients have been treated with this technique; long-term follow-up of patients has ranged from good to excellent. Limitations of tissue engineering include the limited supply of cells and donor site morbidity associated with the initial cartilage harvest. Strategies for developing stem cells for implantation are in the works.

Osiris Therapeutics Inc. (Baltimore, Maryland) is using stem cells derived from bone marrow (i.e., mesenchymal stem cells). These cells are able to differentiate into several of the building blocks of human muscle and bone: osteocytes, chondrocytes, stromal cells or bone marrow matrix, and tenocytes (tendons). Osiris has a large patent portfolio related to the development and application of mSCs. Two products are of particular interest in this area:

- OsteoCel is based on autologous human mSCs delivered on a hydroxyapatite matrix. The product is currently in phase I clinical safety trials involving alveolar ridge generation prior to dental implantation. It is being developed for use in conditions where bones require rejuvenation because of post-fracture difficulty in healing or where sections of bone have been removed following such cancers as osteosarcomas. In preclinical work in dogs, allogeneic mesenchymal stem cells have been used to repair bone.

- Chondrogen uses injectable mSCs suspended in hyaluronan for treatment of meniscus in knee injury.

Geron plans to use human embryonic stem cells for treatment of arthritis. Although arthritis has many causes, the end result is a structural degradation of joint cartilage and a failure of chondrocytes—the cartilage-forming cells—to repair the degraded cartilage collagen matrix. Geron plans to derive chondrocytes from hESCs. If in vitro and animal testing are successful, patients with OA will be treated by injecting the chondrocytes directly into the affected joints.

Diabetes

Diabetes is a chronic metabolic disorder that destroys the body's ability to utilize glucose, a molecule that is very important to all cells. The pancreas produces a hormone called insulin, which regulates the uptake of glucose. When diabetes strikes, β-cells that produce insulin lose their ability to manufacture and release insulin, leading to a build-up of glucose in the blood. Such build-up affects many proteins in the blood and can lead to blindness, kidney failure, and neurological diseases. According to the Juvenile Diabetes Research Foundation, type 1 diabetes (insulin-dependent diabetes) affects an estimated 1.4 million people in the United States; approximately 35 children are diagnosed with the disease every day. The two types of diabetes (type 2 diabetes usually develops later in life and is not insulin dependent) together cause approximately 500,000 deaths in the United States each year.

In 2000 the Edmonton Protocol established a procedure that allowed patients to be transplanted with islets of Langerhans using a specific antirejection drug cocktail. More than 300 transplanted people experienced a dramatic reduction in their need for insulin injections, and some patients no longer required them at all. Transplants of the pancreas have been one solution, but with one million people needing a pancreas transplant and only about 2,000 of the organs available, it is imperative to develop other options.

Dr. S. Kim of Stanford University in California studied 250 diabetic patients who have now been transplanted with islets of Langerhans from cadavers following the Edmonton Protocol. At this time, possibilities for procedures to regenerate replacement islets for type 1 diabetes patients are:

- Pancreatic islet cells
- Pancreatic stem cells
- Embryonic stem cells
- Bone marrow—derived stem cells
- Neural stem cells

Although the idea of using neural stem cells may sound far-fetched, the cells of the endopancreas are derived from the endoderm, not the ectoderm, as are most other organs.

In late 2004, the Singaporean company ES Cell International, which provides products and technologies derived from hES cells, announced a strategic partnership with the Juvenile Diabetes Research Foundation to assist in the development of newly derived nonxenograft human embryonic stem cells (hESCs). The human stem cell islets are developed through the company's proprietary research, which will determine how to convert the islets to conform to the required pharmaceutical quality for widespread use.

Another company, Ixion Biotechnology, Inc. of Alachua, Florida, has developed islet-producing stem cell (IPSC) technology. Using adult pancreases, Ixion can grow functioning stem cell preparations in vitro by isolating IPSCs and culturing, differentiating, and proliferating them before transplanting back into patients. The proof of principle has been shown in a mouse model. When humans receive the treatment, they will be required to take immunosuppressant drugs because the pancreas is from another person. However, Ixion has been working on a second-generation product that will be produced from various tissues from the patient to receive for transplant. Another possibility is using an encapsulated form of allogeneic IPSC in a non-animal hyaluronic acid gel to reduce or eliminate the need for immunosuppressant therapy.

Generally the immune system is thought to be one of the so-called good guys fighting invading enemies like bacteria or viruses or parasites. But sometimes the good guy turns bad, and instead of recognizing foreign bodies from the outside, it turns on its own cells and tissues. When the immune system falters in this recognition, the B and T white blood cells that mediate immunity attack the self-proteins. The result is an autoimmune disease—when the body defenses attack normal tissue.

Rheumatoid arthritis (RA) is one of the autoimmune diseases. About five to eight million people have swollen and disfigured joints because of this condition. The drug methotrexate is a disease-modifying antirheumatoid drug (DMARD), an immunosuppressant that was a major breakthrough of the 1990s. Another groundbreaking therapy is tumor necrosis factor (TNF) antagonist therapy. However, not all patients respond well to these therapies.

On 28 February 2006, Genetech, Inc (South San Francisco, CA). and Biogen Idec (Cambridge, MA) announced the FDA's approval of their therapeutic antibody Rituxan, which is used in combination with methotrexate. Rituxan is the first treatment for RA that selectively targets immune cells known as CD20-positive β-cells. Through the unique mechanism of action, the drug affects the multiple pathways by which β-cells are believed to contribute to the initiation and development of the condition.

Lupus Erythematosus

Systemic lupus erythematosus (SLE) is a multisystem autoimmune disease that, in spite of advances in therapies, continues to cause significant illness and death among patients with active disease. This disease attacks the synovial lining of the joints, producing pain and inflammation, most often in fingers and wrists. It also causes a mask-like rash to appear across the nose and face, giving the look of a wolf to those who suffer from the disease. The word *lupus* is Latin for "wolf"; "erythematosus" has the Greek root *erythemat,* meaning "red." The disease was at one time associated with tales of werewolves, especially because its sufferers are sensitive to sunlight, disposing them to come out only at night. Usually affecting women between the ages of 15 and 35, this lifelong condition causes inexplicable fatigue.

Katherine Hammons was contemplating suicide after two strokes and brain damage as a result of lupus until she entered a study by Dr. Ann Traynor, now at the University of Massachusetts. Traynor used stem cells from Hammons's own bone marrow. Six years after the therapy, her lupus is still in remission and previous damage appears to be healing. Traynor reports that 75 percent of her patients remain in remission from two to eight years after treatment.

Recently, researchers from Northwestern University School of Medicine in Chicago studied patients with SLE who had been resistant to other therapies. *News from the American Medical Association* (2006) reported a trial of 48 patients who underwent treatment with autologous hematopoietic stem cell transplantation (hSCT). The overall five-year survival rate was 84 percent. Stem cells are taken from the bone marrow, grown, and reinfused into patients to make new immune cells. This procedure uses chemotherapy to eliminate defective lymphocytes, after which patients are given the hSCs.

New Organs

Sixteen-year-old Kaitlyne McNamara was born with a condition called spina bifida, in which a part of the spinal column does not close. In addition to 54 surgeries, Kaitlyne is now the possessor of the first engineered bladder. Researchers at Children's Hospital in Boston used a mature progenitor-type cell. They first operated on the patient to remove the bad tissue that composed more than half of her bladder. They fished out muscle and bladder cells; seeded them on a cup-like, bladder-shaped scaffold of collagen; and allowed them to reproduce for seven weeks. They started with tens of thousands of cells and ended up with 1.5 billion cells. Cell-bearing molds were then surgically sewn back to the remnants of the patient's partly working bladder, where the lab-nurtured cells continued to mature.

Burns and Skin Ulcers

Throughout the world, burns and skin ulcers are major causes of morbidity. For decades epidermal skin grafts from parts of victims' bodies have been used. For the last 20 years, techniques of culturing skin stem cells have been used to treat these two conditions. The future for advances in this area looks promising.

Skin is the largest and most exposed organ in the body. It is constantly renewing itself. There are two parts of skin: the epidermis and the dermis. The epidermis is made of layers of epithelial cells, most of which are called keratinocytes, but other cells include Langerhans cells; melanocytes, which give skin its color; and Merkel cells. The epidermis rests upon the dermis, which contains nerve and blood cells that nourish the skin. Epidermal skin cells enable the epidermis to replace itself both in normal circumstances and in traumatic skin loss such as burns and ulcers. Skin ulcers may be caused by several pathological conditions, including diseases, diabetes, and venous ulcer disease. These are difficult to treat because the rate of healing is very slow.

The epidermis is multilayered and continuously renews itself every 30 to 60 days. Most of the activity is restricted to the basal layer, which generates mature functional suprabasal keratinocytes. Epidermal stem cells reside within the basal layer and can self-maintain and self-renew. Keratinocytes are relatively easy to culture and engineer into their normal organ form as sheets of epidermis. Some scientists are convinced that explaining to the public how epidermal stem cells have been used so effectively in health care could be a model for education about stem cells.

Most of the growth of skin tissue in culture for transplants has been from autografts, but there are problems here, including that of time. A few companies are working to develop allografts that may bypass rejection. Lifecell (Branchburg, NJ) has developed Alloderm, a processed human dermis that has the dermal and epidermal cells removed, leaving only the connective tissue matrix. It may be applied to burns and then a cultured autograft may be put on the top of it. Integra (Plainsboro, New Jersey) has produced another dermal substitute made from cow collagen and some synthetic polymers. The ideal bioengineered tissue would be cultured keratinocyte sheets combined with a dermal component containing fibroplasts and other cells. It could be frozen or stored, be inexpensive to make, and give good cosmetic results. These, of course, are not available yet. Culturing autografts takes about three weeks, and is labor intensive and unavailable in parts of the world. Current studies aim to find ways to make the stem cell grow in vitro—as well as in vivo.

Burns often destroy epidermal appendages like hair, sweat glands, and sebaceous glands; thus far no bioengineered equivalents have replaced them. Stem cells within the dermis also have not been successfully cultivated.

Recent work has focused on the hair follicle as a possible source of multipotent stem cells in skin. Dr. D. R. Ma and colleagues in Singapore reviewed the known literature for the location of the stem cells, molecular markers, and multipotency. The stem cells of the hair follicle are located at the bulge region, and the base does contain some cells that will replicate themselves. (See Figure 7.1.) In locating stem cells, markers (or items that may be present to indicate the cells) were present. Some examples of markers are b-1 integrin, keratin 19, and CD34. Using mice and labeling techniques, the scientists found that hair follicle stem cells can repopulate wound epidermis, forming epidermis, hair follicles, and sebaceous glands.

Of course, not all research into stem cells has consequences for medicine. For example, it is not teenagers, the income tax bill, or worry that causes a person's hair to turn gray. The stem cells in the scalp are the culprits. Scientists stumbled across this hair-graying mechanism while they were investigating potential treatments for melanoma, a deadly skin cancer. Stem cells generate melanocytes, the pigment that produces color in the hair and skin. When the stem cells die off with aging or fail to function correctly, the melanocytes go to the wrong place in the hair follicle, and do not create color. However, the scientists said that people should not throw away their cosmetic hair colorings, and that they have no plans to pursue the problem. It is not a top priority.

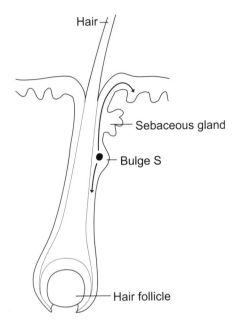

Figure 7.1
Diagram of a hair follicle, illustrating the bulge region. (Illustration by Jeff Dixon.)

Stem cells hold great possibility for therapeutic medicine. Many scientists are working diligently to make it happen. However, the ethical issues of stem cell research continue to dog the process and will not be resolved soon. Section Two considers the complex problems on both sides of the ethical debate, and the regulatory issues that have arisen in many countries.

Ethics and Regulations

Section Two, consisting of Chapters 8 through 13, considers issues related to the ethics and regulation of stem cell research. Both sides are presented. Many of the issues are debated only in medical circles; others are seen every day in the news media. It is not the intent of this book to judge the value of the arguments; rather, it aims to present the debates in a non-biased manner.

First, the issues relating to ethics and religion are presented. Powerful questions are posed in this section:

- What is the meaning of bioethics?
- What are the historical foundations that contribute to understanding stem cell research?
- When dealing with stem cell research, what is ethical and what is right and wrong?
- Is it morally permissible to destroy a human embryo?
- Should we postpone human embryonic stem cell research until all of the controversies surrounding it are addressed?
- Is it acceptable for doctors to experiment on people without their permission if the experimentation is for the common good of humankind?
- Should we create an embryo for a purpose that may destroy it?
- What does informed consent mean?
- When does an embryo become human?
- Should scientists clone embryos?

- What guidelines should govern human embryonic stem cell and therapeutic cloning research?
- How does religion enter into the picture?

Chapter 8 discusses the development of ethical precepts in history and how these principles relate to current problems in stem cell research. Chapter 9 addresses ethical considerations from a twenty-first-century viewpoint, and Chapter 10 considers religion in relation to stem cell research.

Then, the U.S. government's regulation efforts are presented in Chapter 11. Chapter 12 outlines the perspectives on stem cell research in other countries and the consequent development of rules and regulations that may differ from those in the United States. The last chapter, Chapter 13, considers future developments and ethical problems that may occur as our understanding of stem cell research progresses.

Ethics and Research in History

The howling winds of the hurricane beat upon the ship, breaking it into a thousand pieces. Clinging to one floating timber, the sole survivor was happy to see a land of green trees and luscious fruit in the distance. Once on the island, however, he discovered that he was not alone. First he encountered an animal that was a combination of a leopard and a human. Traveling inland, he met the swine-folk (human-pig hybrids). The survivor soon discovered Dr. Moreau, a notorious medical researcher who had been cast out of London for his bizarre experiments.

H. G. Wells's *The Island of Dr. Moreau* is a classic science fiction novel, written in 1896. In the book, Dr. Moreau uses dissection and surgery to create these hybrids, which he called **chimeras,** after the creatures of mythology that were part lion, goat, and serpent.

Scientists today can create chimeras—not with surgery, but with in vitro manipulation. Cells from one species can be inserted into the blastocyst of another species. For example, inserting cells from a goat into the blastocyst of a sheep results in a creature possessing characteristics of both animals, which is called a "geep." Experiments are not limited to animals. Several scientists in different institutions are inserting human cells into a pig to study development at the cellular level.

Science fiction stories like *The Island of Dr. Moreau* and Aldous Huxley's *Brave New World* introduced ethical questions that nineteenth- and twentieth-century readers considered amusing and improbable. Today's readers may have second thoughts as they hear about genetic manipulation of cells and about real chimeras at some research institutions. The questions posed in these fictional stories are real, and the ethical issues they raise are not going away. The challenge is in whether stem cell research can advance to the point where it will be accepted by the public as both scientifically and morally sound.

WHAT IS ETHICS?

Ethics, a discipline of philosophy, deals with what is right and wrong in human behavior and conduct. The word "ethics" comes from the Greek *ethos,* meaning "character." The word "morality" comes from the Latin *moralis,* meaning "customs of manners." Ethics, then, appears to refer to a person's individual character, whereas morality is the relationship between human beings. In everyday life, the terms are used interchangeably.

The term "ethics" also may be applied to specific areas of human life. Bioethics (or life ethics) involves much more than how a doctor treats a patient. It relates to the following areas of medicine: treatment of dying patients, allowing a person to die (mercy death), mercy killing, behavior control, human experimentation, informed consent, genetics, fertilization and birth, population and birth control, **abortion,** organ transplantation, cloning, stem cell research, truth telling in medicine, and confidentiality.

ETHICAL ISSUE: PHYSICIAN, FIRST DO NO HARM

The foundation of our current discussion of the ethics of stem cell research began on the tiny, hilly island of Cos off the coast of Greece in the Aegean Sea. According to legend, Asclepius, the god of medicine, settled his mortal son Podaios on Cos after the Trojan War. All male descendants of Podaios were physicians, known as the Asclepiads. At that time in most of the Greek world, superstition and ritual were parts of the healing tradition. For example, in order to be cured of the illnesses caused by evil spirits, patients would spend a night in the temple, where information about their illness would be revealed by the god of medicine in a dream. The doctors sometimes used harsh treatments even when patients had no chance of recovering. Doctors of the day were considered artisans, so almost any male who desired a career as a physician could become an apprentice.

However, the Asclepiads began to depart from these religious rituals and started a tradition of secular medicine that was based more on observation than superstition. Born about 460 BC on the island of Cos, Hippocrates emerged as an esteemed practitioner of the secular tradition. His methods were gentle, simple, and often effective. He had a deliberate and fatherly concern for his patient and his art. Hippocrates set forth his treatment ideals in his papers thus: "I will give no deadly medicine to anyone if asked, nor suggest any such counsel." In other words, do no harm. This statement becomes very important for those involved in stem cell research. The idea is also binding: never injure one person to benefit another.

About 100 AD Scribonious Largius, a Greek physician, redefined the medical profession in terms of the Hippocratic Oath. The word "oath" originally meant "profession"; followers of a particular profession took an oath and were bound by it. The oath became an official statement that people declared to the tax collector, similar to how today our signature indicates that our income tax returns are correct and prepared to the best of our ability. The Hippocratic Oath made it clear that members of the medical profession have a special obligation to those in their care.

During the Middle Ages, most physicians were ignorant and untrained. Medical practice involved superstitious nostrums and incantations. The Hippocratic corpus (i.e., the collected works of Hippocrates and his followers) reemerged during the Renaissance, along with the rediscovery of other classical texts, and were published in 1525 and 1526. Academic institutions began to teach the Hippocratic ideals and resurrected the practice of having medical students swear to uphold the Hippocratic Oath.

Albert Jonsen (2000), a medical ethicist, argues that the meaning of "do not harm" was a reaction to the tendency to subject patients to the rigors of medicine even though they had no chance of recovering. This did not mean abandonment of the dying patient but rather was a precaution against futile and tortuous therapy. Jonsen also observes that both Eastern and Western cultures used similar ethical precepts: a universal moral atmosphere that surrounds the work of caring for the sick and the use of treatments that work.

For most of the 2,500-year period, medical ethics consisted of physicians defining proper conduct and decorum individually. The level of politeness and respectfulness displayed by a doctor reflected this inner virtue. Until about 1800, professional ethics referred to the doctor's character. A true professional did not need a formal code of conduct; maintaining one's honor and virtue was a sufficient motivator to ensure ethical behavior. But this approach to practice was very individualized and based on one's interpretation of oneself. As such, it was subject to significant abuse.

Thomas Percival (1740–1804) of Manchester, England, first proposed a code of ethics for physicians in 1794. His pamphlet coined the term "professional and medical ethics." This code of ethics gave the medical profession a moral mandate to appraise not only the conduct of individual physicians but also those involved in hospitals and with the distribution of drugs.

Percival's proposal affected code development in America, too. In 1808 the Boston Medical Society developed a code similar to Percival's. When the American Medical Association (AMA) was formed in 1847, the organization's leaders followed Percival's code of ethics. American physician Richard Cabot (1869–1939), who established the discipline of medical social work, was a moral philosopher who recognized that the physician's primary moral duty is to scientific medicine and to the application of that knowledge to the patients for whom he or she cares. Today, graduates of medical schools take the Hippocratic Oath, which states: "I will give no deadly medicine to anyone if asked, nor suggest any such counsel." (See The Oath Written by Hippocrates in Appendix A of this book.)

As knowledge about disease advanced during the nineteenth and twentieth centuries, it became necessary to try more experimental treatments on human beings. Many of the experiments were done without the knowledge or consent of those being treated. Many of the patients died. As the twentieth century progressed, people began to realize that some of these experiments were not proper and questioned the ethics of human experimentation. Concerned with the drastic nature of some of these treatments, they quoted the works of German philosopher Immanuel Kant (1724–1804) and his principle known as **Kant's Practical Imperative.** This ethical principle states that each human being must be considered as a unique end and never used as a means to someone else's end. This means that no human being can be used in trials unless the experiment would be therapeutic for that person and would be no more harmful than treatments normally used for such patients. There should be no experimentation just for the good of humanity or others. If the good is an indirect result, then it is permissible, but the patient must be the primary beneficiary.

Many ethicists follow this guideline and add that experimentation can be done if the person gives informed consent and realizes that, although he or she may not be helped, the experiment may advance scientific understanding. However, when there is doubt that the experiment will further understanding, Kant's Practical Imperative is a good criterion. Kant's argument is at the center of the stem cell controversy because some scientists argue that one must think of the greater good rather than just the individual.

ETHICAL ISSUE: MORAL RULES AND POLITIC ETHICS

The term **deontology** is based on the Greek word for "ought." Deontological principles are based not on consequences or what happens for the good of society, but on the determination of some higher moral standard that guides an individual's actions. A person has a duty to do the right thing. Moral rules come from a higher power, such as God, or from the conscience. In other words, moral rules dictate action. A physician in the community has a duty to behave according to high moral rules. Examples are refusal to take the life of a dying person (i.e., refusal to practice euthanasia) or to perform an abortion. This idea might be called "politic ethics." In history, doctors had many political and ethical decisions to make. For example, should a doctor flee or stay with patients during a Black Death or smallpox epidemic? Today, questions of abortion, informed consent, and the use of embryos as a source of stem cells for medical research require political decisions.

INTRODUCING THE ABORTION ISSUE

In the minds of most people, stem cell research is closely tied to the abortion issue. The term "abortion" is used in many circles without a true understanding of what is happening. Abortion is one of many moral issues with special terms or phrases that need defining.

Definition of Abortion Terms

Abortion. The premature termination of a pregnancy before birth. A *spontaneous abortion* is the same thing as a miscarriage; an *induced abortion* is caused by a woman herself or by another, usually a medical doctor.

Amniocentesis. A procedure performed after the sixteenth week of pregnancy in which a needle is inserted through the uterine wall to withdraw amniotic fluid for study for genetic or other birth defects.

Child. Term used after the fetus is born. The pro-life position refers to the developing human individual as a child from shortly after conception, rather than after birth.

Chorionic villus sampling (CVS). A tool used to diagnose genetic defects in the fetus as early as the ninth week of pregnancy. A flexible catheter extracts some cells from the villi on the chorion, the outermost embryonic layer.

Conceptus. A term meaning "that which has been conceived." Coined by Daniel Callahan (1970), "conceptus" is a neutral term for referring to the developing human and avoids the emotional terms used by the different sides of the abortion issue.

Embryo. The developing human individual from the second through the seventh weeks of gestation or pregnancy.

Fetus. The developing human embryo from the eighth week until birth.

Ultrasonic testing. A noninvasive sound/echo test that is performed by at least 12 weeks to acquire information.

Viability. The state that occurs somewhere between the twenty-sixth and twenty-eighth weeks of gestation, when the conceptus is considered viable, that is, able to survive outside the mother's womb; birth occurs between the thirty-ninth and fortieth weeks of pregnancy.

Zygote. A cell or group of cells that results from the union of sperm and egg cells.

Abortion: An Ancient Procedure

Anthropologists have shown that, from the earliest times, almost all human communities have practiced abortion. Members of some primitive tribes induced abortions by giving pregnant women poisonous herbs or by placing pressure on the abdomen until vaginal bleeding occurred. Abortion techniques are described in the early medical texts of the ancient Chinese and Egyptians. The Greeks and Romans considered abortion a way of maintaining a stable population. Instruments for abortions were uncovered at Pompeii and Herculaneum. Socrates, Plato, and Aristotle suggested abortions, but Hippocrates spoke against it because he feared injury to the woman.

Early Christians condemned abortion before **ensoulment,** the beginning of life in the womb. Like Aristotle, St. Augustine (AD 354–430) believed that the emergence of the fetus came 40 days after conception for a boy and 80 days afterward for a girl. The first reference to abortion as a homicide is contained in the authoritative collection of canon law accepted by the Church in 1140. At the beginning of the thirteenth century, Pope Innocent III wrote that quickening was when a woman first feels the fetus move within her. This moment was when abortion became a homicide; prior to quickening it was a less serious sin. In 1670 an English judge, Sir Matthew Hale, determined that an abortionist was guilty of murder if a woman died as a result of an abortion; no mention was made of the fetus,

Several dangerous abortion techniques were popular in 1803. The drastic techniques led Lord Ellenborough, a British judge, to rule that the abortion of a quick fetus was a capital offense, but abortions performed prior to quickening held lesser penalties. This ruling is significant because it was one of the first on the topic of abortion in British jurisprudence.

From colonial times in the United States to the nineteenth century, the choice of continuing pregnancy or having an abortion was the women's until "quickening." Similar legislative initiatives were passed in the 1820s and were adopted state by state as the frontier moved westward. Not one law had been passed against abortion as of 1800; by 1900 all states had laws banning abortion at any time during a pregnancy. The newly formed American Medical Association influenced laws to take abortion out of the hands of women. In addition, legal barriers to abortion were erected throughout the Western world during the nineteenth century. From the second half of the nineteenth century through World War II, abortion was highly restricted almost everywhere. However, in the 1950s liberalization occurred in some of the countries of Eastern and Central Europe. During the 1960s and 1970s almost all of the remaining developed countries revised their policies.

In the 1960s a coalition of individuals and organizations in the United States, including the AMA, sought to overturn laws and reinstate previous values, which were later embedded in *Roe v. Wade* in 1973. Two basic principles come into conflict in the abortion issue that relate to the stem cell debate:

1. The Value of Life principle addresses both the unborn and the life of the mother.
2. The Principle of Individual Freedom posits that the mother has a right to choose what will happen to her body.

Two powerful questions are involved here:

1. When does life begin?
2. At what point does the unborn fetus deserve the same protection as any other human being?

A corollary of these questions centers on absolute rights. According to the strong antiabortion or pro-life position, the conceptus has an absolute right to life from the moment of conception. The pro-choice position states that women have absolute rights over their own bodies and lives.

When Does One Become Human?

This question—when does one become human—is not new. Philosophers, scientists, and politicians have debated it for over 2,000 years. Aristotle, who always managed to be in on the latest controversy, taught that life existed in three stages: vegetative, animate, and intellectual. While he was probably referring to groups of people, his followers compared it to human development. They argued that humans are in a vegetative state after conception, followed by an animate state, when muscles develop, and ending in the intellectual state. The first two stages took place in the womb and the third after birth. To these Greeks, the embryo did not become human until after birth.

The question about when a person becomes human is integral to the abortion controversy. Three positions shape the ethical arguments related to the beginning of human existence: (1) antiabortion, or pro-life, arguments (called "anti-choice" arguments by some); (2) abortion-on-request, or pro-choice, arguments; and (3) a possible moderate position on abortion. All sides agree that there is life at conception and that from that point it develops along key stages as the conceptus develops. (Refer to Chapter 1.) The reasoning behind each point of view follows.

Antiabortion Arguments

This group believes in the genetic view of the beginning of human life. Life begins at conception. They propose the following points:

- Life is sacred and has value. The right to life is absolute and the innocent unborn children have the same rights as any other human being. Every unborn child must be regarded as a human person from the moment of conception.
- The domino effect may occur if this position is not recognized. For example, Hitler started his history of atrocities by legalizing abortion.
- Abortion is both medically and psychologically harmful to women.
- Modern technological advances negate claims that pregnancy is dangerous for the mother.
- Viable alternatives to abortion exist because unwanted babies can be placed for adoption and because institutions and agencies exist to care for unwanted or deformed children.
- Cost cannot be a factor where human life is concerned.
- Women must take full responsibility for their sexual behavior and cannot sacrifice life because of their carelessness.
- Rape and incest are not problems because contraceptives can often be used in time; rape and incest do not justify taking an innocent life.

Abortion-on-Request: The Pro-Choice Position

This position claims that women have absolute rights over their body and that the conceptus is part of the woman's body until it is born. The following arguments represent this position:

- A conceptus cannot be considered a human being until it is born.
- Unwanted and deformed children should not be brought into the world. It is much more responsible to have an abortion than to bring a child into the world who will be a burden to society. Adoption in this case is not always a solution.
- Abortion is a no-risk medical treatment. There will be more medical and psychological damage to women who go through unwanted pregnancies than to those who have abortions.
- The domino argument of the pro-life movement is not historically accurate. Hitler's allowing abortions is completely different from the reasons that women have abortions today.
- Carrying to term a pregnancy that results from rape or incest is a damaging psychological experience for any woman.
- This choice should be only the woman's; no other person should interfere.

The Moderate Position

This position contends that the strong pro-life and pro-choice arguments cannot be resolved because they are a conflict of absolutes. Its advocates therefore propose the following tenets:

- There are no absolutes for either position. Although the Value of Life principle is important, there is no absolute right to life for the conceptus. On the other hand, although an individual's right to choice is strong, there is no absolute right over one's body and life.
- The point when life begins may be a synthesis of the two positions. The pro-life position draws the line too early (at conception); the pro-choice position draws it too late (at birth).
- The moderate position favors a developmental view of the beginning of life. The conceptus is not human at conception but gains value toward becoming a human being as gestation continues.

Scientists themselves disagree and have varied positions relating to the beginning of life. For example, scientists like Dr. Michael West, CEO of Advanced Cell Technology, believe that cloned human embryos destined for therapeutic research are not really human. Others argue that the Human Genome Project, completed in 2003, leads to a different conclusion.

Scientists have declared for the first time that the human race has access to the information that makes us human. By possessing all the genetic information necessary to be a human, the embryo must be fully human at conception. Similarly, some scientists reject the idea that clones are different from human beings. They argue that clones have the same genetic parts as humans. Dr. Ian Wilmut, the Edinburgh researcher who cloned Dolly the sheep, contends that the clone was a sheep because she had the genome of a sheep. Likewise, it is argued that if a clone has the human genome, it is human, and is human from the day of its conception.

ETHICAL ISSUES: HUMAN EXPERIMENTATION AND INFORMED CONSENT

The revelation of the experiments of Nazi doctors during World War II seared into people's minds just how horrible and inhumane it is to experiment on individuals without their consent. Ethicists pose three justifications for human experimentation: (1) the use of human beings for those persons' own therapy and benefit; (2) participation in trials for the good of humanity in general; and (3) experimentation for purposes of advancing scientific knowledge.

The question arises, why should anyone ever question human experimentation? Animals are wonderful tools for study, but their use can advance medical knowledge about new drugs and procedures only so far. Sooner or later, the drug or technology must be used in humans to determine its effectiveness. Also, some areas of research apply only to humans, and animal experimentation cannot yield the necessary knowledge.

The history of medical research and human experimentation reveals both great successes and horrible abuses. Plagues like smallpox were rampant and capable of wiping out entire cities. People were desperate for relief and would try anything that could help ward off the horrible plagues, even experimenting. English aristocrat Lady Mary Wortley Montague introduced the idea of **variolation** to the gentry in 1715. In variolation, ooze from sores of smallpox victims with mild cases was scratched into the skin. During the French and Indian War, General George Washington was convinced that his most formidable foe was smallpox and he subjected his men to forced variolation to stop its spread. Many of the soldiers had only mild reactions, but some became seriously ill and died. The European press, especially among the antivaccine society, bitterly criticized Washington for forcing his men into possible harm without their consent. Hessian soldiers, who fought alongside the British, were captured and imprisoned in Frederick, Maryland, where they may have been subjected to variolation experimentation—a safety precaution before Washington would order the procedure for his own army. When British physician Edward Jenner (1749–1823) introduced the use of cowpox sores to make a vaccine against smallpox, he was subjected to the same criticism.

In the 1700s principles of individualism, self-determination, and consent of the governed formed the establishment of the United States. Ethicists call this idea the principle of "respect for persons." Therefore, informed consent is a human right and an outgrowth of life, liberty, and the pursuit of happiness.

What Is Informed Consent?

Informed consent is a consequence of the ethical principle of "respect for persons." The person is told about all the possible risks and benefits of a procedure and then considers the intent, action, and consequences of his or her personal decision. However, medical experiments throughout history have been conducted in violation of this principle.

When microbiologists conceived the germ theory of disease, experimenting on people was the only way to learn about causes and prevention. Walter Reed, a famous army doctor and microbiologist, was appointed by the U.S. government to its commission on the study of yellow fever, a scourge during the late 1800s. During the Spanish-American War and the invasion of Cuba, Reed recruited volunteer subjects among soldiers and civilians to test measures for the prevention of yellow fever. He used informed-consent statements written in both English and Spanish to tell the people that risks to the individual were possible if they participated in these experiments.

THE BERLIN CODE OF 1900

As scientific information began to expand around the turn of the twentieth century, ethical questions became important. Berlin microbiologist Rudolf Virchow shared the intense interest in medical ethics that was developing in America. He was concerned about the controversy that broke out in Berlin when German microbiologist Albert Neisser (1855–1916) inoculated unsuspecting subjects with a serum made from the blood of syphilis patients. The Berlin City Council demanded that this practice stop. On the advice of American doctors William Osler and William Welch, Virchow wrote the Berlin Code of 1900 (included in Appendix A).

This code was one of the first and strongest codes governing the ethical conditions to be met before humans could be used in medical research.

However, in 1931 Adolf Hitler signed a memo specifying that this code did not apply to certain groups of people: Jews, gypsies, the mentally disabled, and others. He claimed that such disabled people were not citizens and had no rights. This opened the door for the horrible experiments that took place in the concentration camps of World War II. Thus, in 1947, the Nuremberg Tribunal condemned Nazi doctors for acts of torture, barbarism, and murder rather than acts of medical experimentation. These trials led to the Nuremberg Code for the ethical use of human subjects. According to this code, researchers must meet ten conditions for research involving human experimentation. (The text of the Nuremberg Code is included in Appendix A.)

The U.S. Food and Drug Administration (FDA) began in 1862 with one chemist to analyze the safety of food. However, the Federal Food and Drug Act of 1906 established an agency with the power to approve drugs as well as monitor food safety. In the 1950s the drug thalidomide, which was taken to control nausea during pregnancy, was approved in Europe. A vigilant reviewer at the U.S. FDA kept thalidomide from being approved in the United States. More than 12,000 babies were born with deformities caused by thalidomide, most of them in Europe. In 1962 the Kefauver Amendments were added to the U.S. Food, Drug, and Cosmetic Act to ensure greater drug safety. For the first time, manufacturers had to prove to the FDA that products were effective before marketing them.

The revelation that the U.S. Public Health Service had used indigent black men in Tuskegee, Alabama, to study the effects of syphilis shocked the world. From 1932 until the 1972 exposure of the study, researchers withheld curative treatment in order to study the natural course of the disease. These experiments led to the passage of the National Research Act (PL 93-348) in July 1974, which added restrictions and oversight procedures for research involving human subjects. On 12 July 1975, the American National Research Act created a national commission to identify basic ethical principles governing any research involving human subjects. The commission produced the Belmont Report, named after the Belmont Conference Center at the Smithsonian Institution, where the report was finalized. (The text of the Belmont Report is included in Appendix A.)

The Belmont Report specifies the following ethical principles:

- Respect for persons.
- Beneficence, the natural extension of the Hippocratic Oath that all physicians shall do no harm. Those involved in medical research must never injure one person to benefit another.
- Justice. Those volunteering should receive some benefit from their participation.

- Informed consent. Every participant in a research study must be informed in writing and must receive information in a language that the individual can understand, with instructions that are clearly given.
- Risk/benefit assessment. A formalized method of assessing risk must be in place. Few would volunteer if they thought they would die from their participation. Independent committees must be in place to monitor risks in relationship to the benefits.
- Selection of subjects. Selection must be fair. High-risk experiments should not be performed on just one segment of the population, such as prisoner inmates or members of low-income groups.

The Belmont Report introduced the principle of informed consent. In the United States, the FDA and the National Institutes for Health (NIH) are responsible for enforcing the Belmont Report's guidelines. Local boards called Institutional Review Boards (IRBs) must approve any protocol before experimentation using human subjects may begin. To win approval from the FDA, a drug or procedure must undergo close scrutiny. Stem cell research procedures or studies using human experimentation would fit in this category. See the sidebar Clinical Trials for Medical Research.

Human embryonic stem cell research presents a moral problem that is not normally encountered in research using human subjects, but nonetheless has informed consent implications. The investigator is obliged to protect the donor's welfare. The typical experiment destroys the embryo subject, which raises the question, are embryo-destructive experiments moral?

To many people, the destruction of embryos evokes memories of the experiments done by Nazi doctors. The association does have some merit. Although stem cell research has great potential, and people are calling for increased study in this area, getting the research that may eventually help people with Alzheimer's or Parkinson's disease into the clinic must consider all of the above principles.

It has been more than 50 years since James Watson and Francis Crick announced the decoding of DNA, the genetic code. Their revelation ignited contentious debates that have long captured our collective imagination. Genetic research has raised questions about what we mean by freedom, moral choice, and justice. Human embryonic stem cell research depends on genomics for insight into how cells signal, repress, and express the proteins that shape them. As each piece of the puzzle of genomics is identified, some people see it as threatening the classic disciplines of power and reason. The answer is not a simple one. Chapter 9 frames present ethical issues relating to stem cell research.

Clinical Trials for Medical Approval

After preclinical research, trials are conducted in four phases.

Research Stage	What Happens During the Trials
Preclinical research	Informal experiments are conducted on mice, rats, and monkeys. This is called basic research.
Phase I	After preclinical research, applications are made to the FDA, NIH, and the Recombinant DNA Advisory Committee (RAC) to monitor trials addressing cloning, recombinant DNA, or gene therapy. Phase I trials are small, usually using 2–20 adults who have given informed consent to test for safety.
Phase II	With success in Phase I, investigators use a larger number of subjects (100–300) to continue safety studies but also to study efficacy (i.e., how well the drug works).
Phase III	If Phase II is effective and toxicity is low, investigators recruit thousand of patients at a variety of research centers. This phase is very expensive and time-consuming. If trials are successful, the FDA approves the drug for marketing.
Phase IV	After approval, the drug's performance is monitored for long-term effect, and this follow-up may stretch from 10 to 20 years. The FDA may pull the drug from the market if a problem is uncovered.

Source: Developed by Evelyn B. Kelly.

CHAPTER 9

Ethics and the Brave New World

The students gape as they amble through the nursery. Their assignment is to learn all they can about the Bokanovsky and Podsnap Processes that allow the nursery, called a Hatchery, to produce thousands of identical human embryos. In amazement, they observe the bottles of tiny embryos traveling along a conveyor belt. The instructor explains how the embryos will be conditioned to belong to five groups: Alpha, Beta, Gamma, Delta, and Epsilon. Alpha embryos will become leaders of the World State; deprivation of oxygen and other chemicals will stupefy the Epsilon embryos so that they will be able to perform only menial labor. When Delta infants reach out to grasp a book, or to touch a flower or anything beautiful, they will receive an electric shock. This will teach them never to question anything, and to become easily led, eager consumers.

In this manner does Aldous Huxley open his 1932 novel, *Brave New World.* Books such as *Brave New World* helped agitate the restless undercurrents of distrust and questions about science. The debate heated up again in 1952, when James Watson and Francis Crick announced to the world their discovery of a new molecule, deoxyribonucleic acid (DNA), that was the genetic code of life. Soon, stories and images of genetic manipulation raised questions about the very meaning of freedom, moral choice, and justice as people began worrying that the future might be programmed like the "brave new world." Clearly, the framework of genetic knowledge, or genomics, is essential to understanding how cells work, repress, and express proteins. When Thomson and Gearheart released the stem cell papers in 1998, the same flurry of questions arose anew. Thus, embryonic research became linked to a large arena of social and intellectual debates about the meaning, or *telos,* of the future of humankind, the place of humans in the world, and the very nature of life itself. The resulting debates threatened the power of the classic disciplines of faith and reason.

Ethicists such as Ronald Green (2006) of the Ethics Institute, Dartmouth University, argue that it is the consensus of the scientific community that hES cell research holds great promise for developing treatments for a variety of currently untreatable diseases. However, because it involves the destruction of the embryo, embryonic stem cell research has been the focus of great controversy among the general population. To gain the American public's approbation, scientists and people involved in stem cell research must formulate persuasive answers to ethical questions raised. Likewise, society must address a series of questions in order to translate ethics into accepted public policy. Some individuals encourage postponing the destruction of human embryos until science provides more information about the benefits of adult stem cell research. Others believe that such a delay is not warranted, and that it is scientifically moral to keep both research paths—embryonic and adult stem cell—open.

Laurie Zoloth (2006) of the Center of Bioethics at Northwestern University poses four sets of ethical questions about research:

1. What is the moral status of the embryo? What is the blastocyst and what is one's duty to it? Three positions about the blastocyst may be held:

    -   If one believes that blastocysts are fully human as are newborns, then they merit the respect and protection to which any vulnerable human is entitled. "Ensouled" means that the individual has that spirit of life that renders it human.
    -   If one believes that blastocysts are tissues of worth, such as hearts or kidneys used in transplants, then they deserve care and respect.
    -   If one believes that blastocysts are body tissues, such as the placenta or an amputated limb that can be discarded, then the duty of care and respect is limited to that appropriate to a dispensable human part.

Human eggs are alive; they are not inanimate stones. They have the ability to grow and divide. Biochemical signals tell the early embryo when to turn on certain actions and when to turn them off. Brigid Hogan (2001) pictures the blastocyst as an origami original that needs genetic signals to become properly folded.

Each person must arrive at his or her own answer to the question, is it morally permissible to destroy a human embryo? The issue is deeply entwined with beliefs about abortion, as discussed in Chapter 8. Chapter 10 will look at these issues from religious points of view, and Chapter 11 will explore policy and legal aspects.

2. Can eggs from women be obtained justly All eggs come from specific women; sperm come from specific men. Can gametes coming from couples who desperately want to have children be obtained ethically from the excess eggs of the in vitro fertilization (IVF) process? Some ethicists have raised concerns that women may be manipulated and their bodies exploited to make money by selling their eggs at undue risk to the donor. This concern suggests that women could be valued only for their reproductive capacity. If embryos are made from different parts or various sources, will these modified embryos cheapen the value of life? Would the marketplace begin to demand eggs only from people of high intellect or social status, and discard eggs from those who are physically or developmentally disabled?

3. What will be the long-term consequences of regenerative medicine on the aging process, and for people with disabilities? Some ethicists contend that if the goal of stem cell research is to end human illness and suffering, then that goal is flawed. They believe that dealing with physical and mental illnesses teaches lessons about the meaning of being human. What will happen to compassion for the frail and elderly if the goal of cheerful optimism does not accept disability? Yet others argue that changes would take place progressively over long periods of time, and as research proceeds, the public will accept breakthroughs in incremental steps. At present, nearly all ethicists and researchers are viewing these very early stages of research as hypothetical, and possibilities are still theoretical speculation. The fact is, no cure using stem cell research has been proven.

4. Should scientists share their knowledge of procedures and therapies, or is stem cell research strictly a business venture to achieve fame or fortune?

Such questions have framed debates about conducting just research in a world of injustice.

ARGUMENTS FOR AND AGAINST STEM CELL RESEARCH

Medical and scientific ethicists present arguments for and against stem cell research. These arguments fall into several categories.

Arguments For Stem Cell Research

The arguments for stem cell research described in ethical terms are five: (1) **teleological,** consequential, and **utilitarian** arguments; (2) equivalency arguments; (3) deontological, or duty-based, arguments; (4) arguments from historical precedents; and (5) political arguments.

Teleological, Consequential, and Utilitarian Arguments   Teleological arguments are ethical theories concerned with consequences, actions, or rules. The word "teleological" comes from the Greek word *telos,* meaning "end." The result, or end product, of research is its overriding purpose, and a noble end may justify how it was attained. The goals of research are based on the greatest good for the greatest number, and assume that the greatest good for the majority of people is an optimum outcome. **Consequential** and teleological mean the same thing. Utilitarianism is an ethical theory that states that the value of something is derived from its usefulness. A utilitarian says that an act is right if it is useful in bringing about a good or desirable end for the greatest number of people.

From these points of view, research on stem cells is ethical because it has the potential to achieve great things. The consequentialist and utilitarian envision future therapies that can alleviate human suffering. This viewpoint sees as moral the creation of an embryo to destroy it in order to achieve a beneficial end. In the summer of 2002, the Jones Institute at Norfolk, Virginia, created cells from special lines just to be destroyed. They argued that it is ethically better to use hES cell lines created with the full and informed consent of their donors than to use embryos originally created for reproductive purposes. In addition, with so much attention focusing on research problems and the significant expense of developing new drugs, stem cell cultures that are created solely for this purpose would enable pharmaceutical companies to conduct tests for toxicity in humans that cannot be accomplished with animal experiments.

Utilitarian and teleological points of view lead to the issue of cloning embryos. Human **therapeutic cloning** is the deliberate creation of a clone using somatic cell nuclear technology. If people have embryos cloned from their own skin cells or other cells, the spare embryos made to order would get around the problem of immunological rejection. The cloning subjects would have a host of cells that were identical to their own cells.

The creation of clones raises another question: is the clone a human embryo in the accepted sense of the term? Clones could be used to counter the argument of those who believe that life begins at conception, because nuclear transfer is not fertilization. Another speculative problem arises: if the technique of cloning becomes very technologically advanced, or even perfected, then how long will it be before children are cloned? The broad consensus in the scientific community is that cloning poses serious physical and psychological risks to a child created in this way. Cloned animals evidence many physiological problems, and tend to die early.

Another argument for stem cell research is that it permits the study of genetic diseases at the cellular level. Devotees of this position believe that research should embrace a fully open *telos* as principled scientific policy.

Equivalency Arguments   This form of argument compares stem cell research to other research being done in medical centers in approved in vitro fertilization procedures. In fertility clinics, many eggs are injected with sperm, given growth factors, and used as teaching tools for physicians learning to perform the IVF procedure. Institutional Review Boards (IRBs) have approved this experimentation, and embryos are destroyed at 14 days, just before they form the primitive streak. Embryos are created with the understanding that few will survive. Approved procedures for IVF have called for implanting up to eight embryos in the uterus in the hope that not all will die. If more than three embryos do implant, then the couple is offered embryo reductions, which means selective abortion.

Deontological, or Duty-Based, Arguments   In ethics, the term "deontological" refers to duty-based reasons to perform an action. For example, people vote and are good citizens because it is their duty to do so. Doctors may heal the sick with compassion because it is their professional duty. Duty-based arguments may spring from a sense of religious duty, in response to a command from God. People who argue from this point of view believe that because there is so much suffering in the world, support of stem cell research is their moral duty.

Arguments from Legal and Historical Precedents   This form of argument asserts that the majority is right. If the majority believe that certain actions are proper, then progress demands moving ahead, in spite of the dissenting minority, such as minority groups who disagree with wars or protest against a movement. Sometimes, it is necessary to move ahead for what is right. These proponents argue that if the majority of people support stem cell research, then it should become public policy, although a loud minority may disagree and protest.

Political Arguments   If research is not publicly supported, then private enterprise may support research that is more questionable or that would benefit only a segment of the population. For example, the trend in private research is to develop pharmaceuticals for profit rather than to benefit people with "orphan drug" conditions; a prominent example is the focus on money-making Viagra, rather than pediatric medicines. Governmental control would supervise activity and prevent undesirable, rogue activity.

Arguments Against Stem Cell Research

The arguments against stem cell research contend that such research is immoral, and that stopping it is righteous and necessary. Arguments against stem cell research also fall into five major categories: deontological, or duty-based, objections; teleological objections; slippery-slope arguments; feminine and environmental objections; and concerns with scientists.

Deontological Objections   This point of view argues that embryonic stem cell research requires the murder of emerging human beings and is morally reprehensible. America's social contract demands protection of the most vulnerable, even a blastocyst. Using the embryo as a tool of research cheapens the value of human life. It is unreasonable to anticipate that all human suffering can be alleviated, and suggesting that aging and suffering can be eliminated devalues compassion for those who are frail and vulnerable.

Teleological Objections   What will be the result of all this stem cell research? Supporters of the teleological argument against such research say that we have no idea where the research may end, and how many people will be hurt in the experimentation. Views of a "brave new world," with social engineering, designer babies, or perfect people, are repugnant to proponents of this position.

Slippery-Slope Arguments   A person may be climbing a mountain looking to reach the top, but lose his or her footing on loose rock and slide downhill. The "slippery-slope" argument suggests that we have no idea where stem cell research will lead. Opponents point to the American and German eugenics experiments before World War II, in which those who were ill or frail were targeted for sterilization in the name of benefiting mankind. Manipulation of embryos could lead to the same thing. The government, or others, could determine whose life is valuable and whose is not. Some fear that cloning will lead to classes of humans, or chimeric human-animal monsters as depicted in *The Island of Dr. Moreau.*

The slippery-slope proponents point to the ethical dilemma that arises with regard to testing human brain cells in primates. If stem cells are ever to be proven therapeutic, they must first be tested in animals. Nicolas Wade (2005) reported in a *New York Times* article quoting the journal *Science* that a group of scientists and ethicists are advising researchers to exercise care, especially if they envision using a large portion of human neurons. Dr. Ruth Faden of the Bioethics Institute at Johns Hopkins believes that monkeys and apes should not be used in experiments. Introducing numerous neurons into the brain of a chimpanzee, she theorizes, could possibly alter the cognitive ability of the animal, making it less of a chimpanzee and more like a human being. Ergo, this kind of experiment could produce an ethical dilemma. Faden has recommended guidelines to the FDA for experimenting with higher-order animals like primates.

Feminine and Environmental Justice   The feminine argument holds that women may be exploited as embryo farms to provide eggs for stem cells. Money that could be spent for prevention and treatment for all segments of society would be spent on this research. Those concerned with environmental aspects worry that experimenting with the human gene pool may cause problems similar to what has happened in nature with species such as the Florida panther, now on the verge of extinction.

Concerns with Scientists   Another troublesome question is, can scientists be trusted? Those raising this question believe that scientists should not be trusted to play God, and because research activities are difficult to monitor and regulate, nothing less than a complete ban on stem cell research is acceptable.

University of Michigan researcher Raymond DeVries (2006) published a study that echoed this sentiment. He cites perhaps a dozen incidents each year of serious misconduct that call into question the integrity of science. He believes that the competitive nature of research fosters an environment in which scientific misbehavior is more prevalent than suggested by just those cases that make headlines. Using both qualitative and quantitative methods, his team found the behaviors apparently most threatening to be common disagreements as to the meaning of data, the rule of science, life with colleagues, and the pressure to produce. Possibly, the issue with South Korean scientist Woo Suk Hwang is only the tip of the iceberg.

IS THERE A COMPROMISE AND POSSIBLE ANSWER?

Zoloth contends that ethicists are good at raising questions and describing the pro and con positions, without putting forth positive suggestions. She recommends several points for consideration:

- Create a range of civic responses that will regulate research—more than just red light/green light responses that prohibit abuse or coercion. Each project needs assessment, rather than merely those that get a lot of publicity.

- Research should be funded, encouraged, and rewarded.
- The process should be more fully explained to the public so people will come to understand that all research is risky, and that failure and error are always possible. The public must be taught patience.
- A public oversight committee could make a strong contribution to the resolution of the basic controversy.
- A moral agency for debate could investigate the issues of relationships between researchers and donors, and how this research shapes us as a society.

Medical ethics has given way to bioethics, a word invented in the 1960s to encompass the newly created world of experimental biology. Today, medical ethics is an academic discipline, with a distinct literature and experts who specialize in the subject. When medical ethics first developed, the physician was the one who decided what was right or wrong. Codes of ethics to weed out imposters and charlatans developed to help address the behavior of doctors in their practices. The concept of respect for the individual, and the idea of each individual taking some responsibility for his or her own health, are relatively new elements in the discipline. Another item that might now be added to the body of medical ethics is the use of empirical data to help answer questions. Bioethics will continue to change and evolve as discoveries, especially those relating to the critical area of stem cell research, are made. Knowing the past can enlighten the future.

CHAPTER 10

Religious Considerations

Two scientists were discussing faith and beliefs. One was a committed atheist, bitter about what he perceived as the deception of the church in leading people to live by their emotions. The other scientist was a conservative Christian, who believed that there is no conflict between faith and science, and that guidelines for ethical behavior must come from precepts in the Bible. Obviously, the two had little common ground for understanding each other's points of view. This illustration only hints at the disputes that arise when religion enters into the debate about stem cell research.

Religious faith offers people hope to make sense out of their lives. Religion is powerful because it addresses topics such as death, suffering, hope, history, community, and precepts for everyday living. Although many groups have common religious traditions, great variations of beliefs exist among various groups, as well as within traditions that bear similar names. Probably no area engenders such broad religious disagreement as stem cell research. For example, Roman Catholics may not agree with Jewish spokespersons about the nature of abortions. Among Protestant groups, there are vast differences in the positions of the United Church of Christ and the Southern Baptists.

QUESTIONS OF SOURCES AND NATURE

Stem cells themselves are not the center of the dispute; rather, it is the source of the stem cells. The moral status of the embryo and the question of when life begins are the basic concerns. Chapter 9 defined three positions: If one believes that blastocysts are fully ensouled as are newborns, then they are due the respect and protection due any vulnerable human. If one believes that blastocysts are tissues of worth, such as a heart or kidney to be used in a transplant, then they deserve care and respect. If one believes that blastocysts are body tissues such as a placenta or an amputated limb that can be discarded, then one's duty is the care and respect appropriate only to a dispensable human part. All religious thinkers do agree that the embryo deserves respect, even if not in equivalent form or to the same degree. Of course, the exact definition and interpretation of "respect" are not clear.

Religious thinkers who hold the first position, that the fertilized embryo is a human being and deserves protection, will consistently oppose the extraction of stem cells because the embryo must be killed to obtain these cells. Those who do not consider the embryo a viable human person will be more willing to favor embryo and stem cell research. Others who are uncertain as to the nature of the embryo may consider that the benefits of research outweigh any possible violations of the nature of the embryo.

Most religions recognize that aborted fetuses are dead; however, those that prohibit abortion consider the procedure a moral evil, and therefore obtaining stem cells from this source is not acceptable. These religious traditions may support alternative sources, such as adult cells, provided that the donors are not harmed. At the same time, these traditions may also object to the use of existing stem cell lines. Nearly all religious groups agree that buying and selling human embryos is not proper, and that informed consent from donors is essential.

Both secular and theological thinkers ponder stem cell issues as they relate to justice. Questions arise as to who will be the primary donors of embryos or aborted fetuses, and whether race, gender, and class will dominate the process of stem cell research. Will profit enter in? Who will gain from the advances in stem cell research? : Will only the rich benefit from scientific advances? The rich and the poor? Both secular and religious ethicists ponder the questions that were posed in Chapter 9, but religious thinkers refer to the scriptures and the moral reasoning of their faith for guidance. Traditions of each faith concerning stem cells are complex, but appear to be becoming more solidified as research progresses.

RELIGIOUS TRADITIONS AND STEM CELL RESEARCH

To understand religious positions relating to stem cell research, one must examine some of the basic tenets of the major faiths. Not all faiths can be included, and others may hold express positions. Several of the world's major religious traditions—Buddhism, Hinduism, Islam, Judaism, Roman Catholicism, and Protestantism—are considered here.

Buddhism

Siddhartha Gautama, the Buddha, or teacher, lived in the sixth century BC and taught that one must strive for a state of mind called nirvana. Nirvana is not a specific set of beliefs, but a transcendent state where the reality of things is understood and suffering is extinguished. One comes to this state through meditation. Buddhists do not worship a single, omnipresent, all-knowing god as do adherents of many religions. Modern Buddhists are action-centered, rather than worship-centered, and practice a simple regimen of self control and humility, a dedication that outweighs commitments to ritual and religious law.

Thinkers from Buddhism have not generally been major players in the stem cell debate, although some of the countries where Buddhist traditions are strong have been world leaders in developing stem cells. South Korea and Singapore are notable among these countries (as discussed in Chapter 12). Buddhist spokespersons have not articulated a position, but beliefs and traditions about the value of life and the nature of human beings are inherent in the faith.

Hinduism

The traditions and beliefs of Hinduism are complex, and appear conflicting at times. According to Hindu traditions, human life begins prior to conception, and the soul may exist in sperm. In Hindu beliefs, medicine comes to humans as divine knowledge, and it must conform to the divine will. The sacred texts, the *Upanishads,* discuss reincarnation and karma, the belief that all actions produce consequences for the future. Through meditation, devotion, and good works, the individual readies himself for reincarnation, and ultimately to achieve unification with the universal being, or Brahman. Dharma, the right path to salvation, is attained by following certain commandments; high moral demands are placed on believers.

The problem of reincarnation complicates what may be done with embryos. Incarnation offers the opportunity to influence the future of the individual, and the person must live a life emphasizing compassion toward others. Hindu tradition includes nonviolence, but there is also a tradition of sacrifice, where one human life may be taken for a higher cause. This "higher cause" rationale may embrace embryonic stem cell research.

Islam

Teachings of the prophet Muhammad are written in the *Qur'an,* or *Koran.* Hadiths supplement and explain the teaching of the Prophet. Many schools of thought exist among Muslims, and Muslim philosophies range from moral realism to divine command.

Margaret A. Farley (2006) of Yale Divinity School in New Haven, Connecticut, told of the testimony of Islamic scholar Abdulaziz Sachedina before the U.S. National Bioethics Committee in 1999. Invoking various Islamic traditions, he analyzed texts to infer guidelines on the moral status of the embryo. In different eras, perceptions of the early embryo have varied, but legal rulings have determined a developmental view of the fetus according to a divine plan. This suggests that the personhood of the embryo does not exist in the earliest stages, but only after certain stages of biological development have taken place. Most Sunni and Shi'ite scholars recognize two stages of pregnancy: the first before ensoulment, and the second at the time of quickening, at about 120 days. It is at the point of quickening that the biological human becomes a person. During the first stage, abortion is permitted for proper reasons; after the fourth month, abortion is considered homicide. With this in mind, Islamic thought may present justification for embryonic stem cell use without violating divine laws.

Judaism

The three branches of Judaism—Orthodox, Conservative, and Reform—take different positions on many issues of applied ethics. Jewish law does not give legal status to the fertilized ovum outside of the mother's uterus. When the embryo is in the uterus it has legal rights, but not those of a human being. Reform Judaism is probably the clearest supporter of stem cell research from embryos or aborted fetuses.

Farley describes the theological assumptions of Rabbi Elliott Dorff relating to stem cell research:

- Moral discernment of what God wants for his people must be based on both Jewish theology and Jewish law.
- All humans are created in the image of God and must be valued as such.
- Human bodies belong to God and are only on loan to the individuals who reside in them.
- Human response to illness can be natural or artificial.
- There is a duty to develop and use any therapies that can help in the care of the human body.
- Human beings are not God, and humility and caution must be used when science and technology press to the edge of human knowledge.

Jewish thought appears to support the idea that the fetus is like the thigh, a part of the mother. Jewish law possibly permits derivation of stem cells from both aborted fetuses and human embryos. Although generally forbidden, abortion can be justified for serious reasons; so, then, can the use of fetuses for important research. Testifying before the National Ethics Bioadvisory Committee, Rabbi Moshe David Tendler explained that, in Jewish law and tradition, the embryo has no moral status until 40 days after implantation. Until a child is born, it is viewed as a part of the mother's body. Eggs and sperm mixed in a petri dish have no legal status until they are implanted in the mother's womb. Thus, during the first 40 days after implantation, they are only like water, and are non-souled.

Jewish scholars believe that humans have a responsibility to the community to alleviate suffering, and that stem cell research may enable such an outcome. However, they also agree that one must be cautious not to link stem cell research with programs of eugenics.

Roman Catholicism

Aristotle held the view that life begins 40 days after conception. In early Christian traditions, Augustine of Hippo and Thomas Aquinas adopted the Aristotelian position, which was maintained for centuries. In 1869 the view that one cannot know with certainty when life begins supplanted the old view, and the Roman Catholic Church currently holds the belief that the beginnings of life occur at fertilization.

Although many points of view are presented, Catholic tradition is undivided in the goodness of creation, the role of human persons as agents, and the importance of the individual and the community. The debate relating to stem cell research among Catholic theologians appears to relate primarily to the 14-day theory. The theorists look to the reality of stem cells and their sources, and admit that not all the answers are in the Bible or official church teachings. The argument against acquiring stem cells from human embryos is that this causes the death of the embryo. While no one disputes the necessity of the death, the disagreement focuses on whether this can be justified. Those holding the position that death of the early embryo cannot be justified contend there is an **ontological** continuum from the single cell to birth, through life, and then to death. They refer to the fact that each individual has a new and complete genetic code after fertilization, and that a unique individual then exists. If the embryo has the status of a person, then killing it cannot be justified.

Some Catholic theologians hold to the beliefs supported by Aristotle and Thomas Aquinas—referred to as Aristotelian and Thomistic doctrine—and do not consider the human embryo in the earliest stages to be a human person, either potential or actual. Australian Catholic moral theologian Norman M. Ford supports the view that an early embryo is not a potential human person because it is not yet a "self-organizing organism." He contends that the individual is realized in about 14 days, when the being is becoming organized. Until that time cells are totipotent, and can become any part of a human being, or even a whole human being. Ford believes that fertilization is not the beginning of the development of the human being, but the beginning of a formative process.

G. R. Dunstan (1984), an Anglican theologian, claims that absolute protection for the human embryo from conception is a recent stand in Roman Catholic moral tradition. He contends that the position is a novelty, created in the nineteenth century. He believes that the Hebrew beliefs of when the soul enters the body came out of the civilization of the Levant, a group of people who influenced Old Testament laws. Another group of people who influenced Hebrew thinking were the Hittites, who based penalties for assault on pregnant women on the gestational age of the fetus. Later cultures of the region made similar distinctions relating to abortion. However, by the mid-nineteenth century, advances in medicine were making abortion by direct assault on the fetus possible and safer, causing the incidence of abortion to rise. Pope Pius IX ordered excommunication for all who procured abortions, and made no distinction as to method or gestational age.

The two opposing Catholic views continue to be debated. The 1974 Declaration on Procured Abortion states in a footnote that the question of the moment when the spirit (or soul) is infused remains open. Pope John Paul II made no decision on the question of delayed ensoulment in his 1995 encyclical letter. Both sides do agree on the dignity of human life, and the honor of sacred creation.

Protestantism

While diversity and pluralism exist among the many Protestant denominations, the common thread of divine revelation in the person of Jesus Christ, the goodness of creation, and the need for compassion and justice predominates in their beliefs. Their doctrines do not appear to address stem cell research.

Southern Baptists, as a group, do not support embryonic stem cell research, although they consider a possible compromise in the use of already harvested cells. Some leaders of the United Methodist Church have asked President George W. Bush to oppose federal funding for cells extracted from embryos.

Ethicists from various denominations—although usually not speaking for their groups—also vary in their approach to stem cell research. Ted Peters of the Pacific Lutheran School of Theology supports embryonic stem cell research because he believes that the value of human dignity outweighs the dignity of the embryo. Ronald Cole-Turner of the United Church of Christ approves the extraction of stem cells from embryos, but sets conditions for research in terms of justice issues.

Evangelicals and Roman Catholics have engaged in prominent debates about stem cell research. Many Evangelicals and many Roman Catholics oppose the derivation of stem cells from embryos. The 14-day position is a possible, though unlikely, alternative for these groups.

Religious debates over embryonic research probably will not subside in the near future. The question of when the embryo is ensouled and becomes human is entwined with the abortion debate, and neither debate will soon be resolved. While most religious faiths do support adult stem cell research, once the ethical questions presented in Chapter 9 are addressed, some compromise with regard to embryonic research may be achieved. Perhaps if major breakthroughs come in the adult stem cell area, or other ways of producing stem cells materialize (as discussed in Chapter 13), Americans who hold strong religious values may accept the expansion of stem cell research. However, compromise probably will come neither easily nor soon.

CHAPTER 11

Regulatory Issues in the United States

Legal brief: Roe v. Wade

Plaintiff: Using the name "Jane Roe," Norma McCorvey represented all pregnant women in a class action suit.

Defendant: Henry V. Wade, Dallas County, Texas, district attorney.

Plaintiff's claim: The Texas abortion law violated the rights of McCorvey and other women.

Justices: Harry Blackmun (who wrote the opinion for the majority), William Brennan, Chief Justice Warren Burger, William O. Douglas, Thurgood Marshall, Lewis Powell, and Potter Stewart, all on the majority side; William Rehnquist and Byron White, dissent.

Place: Washington, D.C.

Date of decision: 22 January 1973.

Decision: Invalidated all state laws restricting abortion and women's access to abortion during the first trimester of pregnancy, and upheld those second-trimester restrictions that protected the health of pregnant women.

Significance: The landmark decision made abortion legal in the United States.

See Appendix A for the full text of *Roe v. Wade*.

In 1879 the state of Texas passed a law that made abortion a criminal offense except to save the mother's life. This law had stood for nearly a century, with similar laws in other states, when Norma McCorvey, 21, became pregnant in the summer of 1969. Her marriage had failed and she did not want to continue her pregnancy. She could not find someone to perform an abortion, but she did meet Sarah Weddington and Linda Coffee, two attorneys interested in changing the abortion law. McCorvey agreed to become "Jane Roe" in an upcoming test case. After several years of legal maneuvering, the case, known as *Roe v. Wade,* was heard by the U.S. Supreme Court. On 22 January 1973 the Supreme Court announced its decision, which was that the state could not restrict the right of a woman, in accord with her doctor, to obtain an abortion during the first trimester of pregnancy. The court said that states could make laws regulating the safety of abortion procedures as they affected maternal health and that the state could prohibit abortion during the third trimester when the fetus was viable.

In the early 1970s, the ruling reflected thought among some pundits that a liberal attitude toward abortion was prevalent and that the majority of people would accept the ruling without question. This perception turned out to be wrong. The members of the Court had affirmed that the fetus is not a person, and as state lawmakers began to ponder the question, millions expressed their dissatisfaction. By the mid-1970s abortion had become *the* hot topic, one with deep moral implications. Abortion brought to light the ethical questions of when life begins and when a human comes into being.

With the birth in 1978 of Louise Brown, the world's first baby born as a result of in vitro fertilization, and with the success of in vitro reproductive technology in the late 1970s, debate resumed along the slippery slope of where this knowledge might be leading. Nearly two decades later, when scientists announced that cloning had produced a living mammal—Dolly, the sheep—the debate over the moral implications of science ignited into a rampaging fire. With the later announcement that two scientists had created stem cell lines, abortion and embryonic stem cell research became connected in many people's minds.

One of the most prominent examples of this connection is the three-decade debate about the source of funding for any type of research that creates or destroys human embryos or for the use of these embryos in scientific research. Immediately after *Roe* in 1973, some members of Congress became concerned about the possibility of using aborted fetuses in research. In response, the Department of Health, Education, and Welfare (HEW), the precursor of today's Department of Health and Human Services (HHS), issued a moratorium on the use of embryos or fetuses in research. In 1974 Congress enacted the policy into law and initiated a temporary moratorium on federal funding for clinical research using live human fetuses before or after induced abortion unless the research was done for the purpose of studying survival mechanisms of the fetus. Congress also established the National Commission for the Protection of Human Subjects of Biomedical and Behavioral Research to set guidelines for human fetal and embryonic research so that standards for funding could be established and the blanket moratorium might be lifted.

The Commission issued its report in 1975 and the statutory moratorium was lifted. The report called for establishing a national Ethics Advisory Board (EAB) within HEW to propose standards and research protocols for funding of research using human embryos. Because the first successful in vitro fertilization (IVF) in animals was announced in 1969, the Commission realized it needed to consider what would happen if IVF were to be accomplished in humans.

When news of the first test tube baby hit the papers in 1978, Congress finally acted to create an Ethics Advisory Committee (EAC) to apply guidelines for research in this area. The EAC issued an opinion concerning in vitro embryos in its report dated May 1979. The Committee concluded that research involving embryos was ethical provided that the research did not take place after 14 days of development and that all gamete donors were married couples. The report recommended support for a gamut of research projects using human embryos and even for the deliberate creation of embryos for therapeutic research. But release of this report created a firestorm of response from the public. The committee received nearly 13,000 letters—all but 300 of which opposed in vitro fertilization research. The Committee had not advised HEW about how much of the research would be federally supported or how much funding the research should receive. No action was ever taken on the report because after Joseph Califano, Jr., Secretary of Health, Education, and Welfare, resigned in September 1979, no other HEW secretaries took up the issue. When the charter of the Ethics Advisory Board expired in 1980, no channel existed to review proposals for federal funding; thus, during the 1980s no action was taken, and a de facto moratorium on research on embryos was maintained through the Reagan and Bush years. However, research on infertility and embryos did continue with the use of private funds.

THE CLINTON ADMINISTRATION

When William Jefferson Clinton took office in 1991, his administration had a new outlook on reproductive medicine. Supporters of infertility research at the National Institutes of Health (NIH) encouraged Congress to pass legislation that nullified the requirement that the EAB approve federal funding for in vitro and embryo research. This act was called the

Revitalization Act of 1993 or PL 103-43. For the first time in 15 years, NIH was free to fund research proposals in this area. The NIH soon saw that there was a need for guidelines to instruct members of Institutional Review Boards (IRBs), which control human subject research. To give guidance to these local institutions, the NIH formed the Human Embryo Research Panel.

The current stem cell controversy began in 1998 with the publication of research in two prestigious scientific journals. James Thomson of the Wisconsin Primate Center and John Gearhart of Johns Hopkins University published in *Science* and *Nature* articles on stem cell research using two different methods: (1) one in which cells are taken from the inner cell mass of very early embryos; and (2) one that uses cells from the gonadal ridges of aborted fetuses. The work prompted great excitement and led to interesting speculation and research in the United States and abroad. It also sparked a moral and political debate about federal support for such research. Proponents of federal legislation asked whether it is moral to withhold support from research that holds such human promise. Opponents questioned whether it is right to publicly support research that depends on the exploitation and destruction of human life, even if it might be beneficial.

Ronald M. Green (2001), professor of ethics at Dartmouth University, was one of 19 members to serve on the Human Embryo Research Panel. Green told how the committee was given a crash course in in vitro fertilization, including how embryos were graded for implantation. They were concerned that no one had a clear idea of what made a good egg or bad egg and that this poor understanding had serious implications for reproductive medicine. The panel expressed the fear that instead of doing research for understanding, physicians were concerned about making the IVF work, possibly creating risks. The panel pondered such questions the moral status of the embryo, the issue of research embryos, and cloning. But with such a panel, controversy is only a moment away. Green recounts how on 21 June 1994 he was surprised to find a small stack of papers with the top page reading *The Michael Fund et al. v. Ronald M. Green.* He was being sued by The Michael Fund, a support group for persons with Down syndrome, which had instituted an injunction to stop the work of the panel because it would take away funds from research that could go toward Down syndrome. The suit was later dismissed as frivolous; but Green described how the work of the panel ended with a new "Ice Age," or freeze, on embryonic research when a more conservative Congress was elected in 1994.

In 1993 Congress enacted the NIH Revitalization Act, which held that research protocols did not have to be approved by an Ethics Advisory Board. This Act opened the door to the possibility of NIH funding for human embryo research using IVF embryos. The NIH convened a Human Embryo Panel to propose guidelines and concluded that the creation of human embryos with the explicit intention of using them only for research purposes should be very limited. President Clinton overruled the panel on the recommendation of any creation of embryos for research, but he accepted the panel's recommendation that the NIH consider applications for funding research using leftover embryos from IVF procedures.

THE DICKEY AMENDMENT

Congress did not agree with Clinton's recommendations and in 1996 prohibited funds for any research. The amendment was known as the Dickey Amendment, named after Representative Jay Dickey (R-AR), who wrote the amendment. The two key points of this provision are that no funds shall be used for either of the following:

- The creation of a human embryo for research purposes
- Research in which a human embryo is destroyed, discarded, or knowingly subjected to injury or death

The prohibitions were for federally funded research and did not apply to research using private funding.

The isolation of embryonic stem cells in 1998 caused quite a stir in the research communities. The research had been supported in large part by private funds, and some questioned the policy of withholding federal funds from human embryo research. But most members of Congress did not change their positions, and the Dickey Amendment has been renewed every year.

In 1999 the General Counsel of the Department of Health and Human Services argued that the wording of the law might permit the interpretation that it would be legal to use federal funds for human embryonic stem cell research. If researchers using private funds first destroyed embryos, then later performed research using cells that were propagated in these tissue cultures, they might be eligible for federal funding; the legal requirement would still technically be obeyed. Some argued that while this may fit the letter of the law, it did not reflect the spirit of the law. Others said that promoting this research, especially with its potential for therapy, was an obligation of government.

The Clinton administration supported this course of action and drew up specific guidelines to enact it, but it was never put into practice.

THE BUSH YEARS

In July 2001 the U.S. House of Representative passed the Human Cloning Prohibition Act, H.R. 2505, which prohibited human cloning in all forms. The bill had broad-based support in the House, but the Senate opposed the bill, and it was defeated. The major points of contention came from patient advocate groups who agreed to ban reproductive cloning but argued in favor of therapeutic cloning. The bill never became law, but in 2003 it was reintroduced. The House approved it by a margin of 241 to 155, but it stalled again in the Senate.

On 9 August 2001 George W. Bush made his first major public policy address broaching the topic of federal funding for human stem cell research. He announced that after several months of deliberation, he had decided to make federal funding available for research involving only certain lines of embryo-derived stem cells. The text of this speech and the registry listing the stem cell lines that were accepted are included in Appendix A.

Bush also declared his intention to name a President's Council to monitor stem cell research, to recommend appropriate guidelines and regulations, and to consider all of the medical and ethical ramifications of biomedical innovations.

The Council on Bioethics reviewed the background on why there is public contention about stem cell research in a 2004 report. They agreed that most people support research; the problem is the ethical issue of how the cells were obtained. Most of the argument pertains to what to do with spare embryos after IVF enters clinical practice. Although research using these embryos has not been illegal except in a few states, the federal government has never funded it, and since 1995 legislation has prohibited the use of taxpayer dollars for research where human embryos are harmed or destroyed.

WHY NEW EMBRYONIC CELL LINES?

Embryonic stem cells and embryonic germ cells are not embryos or whole organisms. They cannot be made into organisms. They have been derived and grown in a laboratory culture; no other cells will be destroyed to work from that line. The problem arises from the uncertainty as to whether these lines can persist indefinitely, and only a limited number of lines have been made. Scientists believe that developing new lines is desirable, and many cells are cryopreserved now as a potential source of stem cells. Complicating the issue is the use of a group of tissues called adult stem cells, which does not involve destroying embryos. Some people believe that adult stem cells alone are sufficient for research and study.

Large commercial interests have already invested in stem cell research in the United States and throughout the world, and such research continues to grow as a business venture. Chapter 13 takes a look at the future of stem cell research.

Other questions also arise. Should moral considerations be used to decide what sort of research may or may not be funded? What is the symbolic, moral, and political significance of procuring national approval? Conversely, what are the symbolic problems of doing nothing? Are there premature claims about the great promise of stem cells that are not scientifically substantiated, and do these claims exploit sick people and their families, giving them false hope? Some advocates have made bold claims about the number of people who could be healed with the research. Is this hyperbole, aimed at playing on the hopes and fears of the public? The value of therapeutic cloning is more difficult to sell in the United States because the abortion issue has polarized the country much more than in the UK.

The Council's task of monitoring stem cell research issues is like watching water flow over Niagara Falls. Reports pour forth daily, and sometimes it is difficult to separate hope from hype.

CURRENT FEDERAL LAW AND POLICY

The Bush policy has been misunderstood and at times misrepresented by both its detractors and advocates. Whether one agrees with the policy or not, it is important to understand what has been said and place it in its proper context.

Each year the federal government makes significant resources available to biomedical researchers. In 2003 over $20 billion was offered in the form of grants, mostly from the National Institutes of Health (NIH). Those who accept the funding must abide by certain ethical rules and regulations, especially regarding the use of human subjects for research. Some policymakers and citizens have always insisted that tax dollars must not be invested in research that violates the moral beliefs of portions of the American public. At times the concern for the moral sensibilities of taxpayers has led to disputes over federal funding.

In 2001 President Bush stated that he wanted a way to allow valuable research to proceed while upholding the spirit and not just the letter of the Dickey Amendment.

The Dickey Amendment still rules. The logic of the moral and political understanding behind the Amendment still forms the foundation of the current policy. When the policy was announced, numerous stem cell lines already existed and were in various phases of growth, and these embryos were already dead. Bush put it this way in 2001: Life and death decisions had already been made. Those decisions made it possible to use taxpayer funding for research only on those preexisting lines.

From the moment of the announcement, the policy has been hotly contested. It reflects a desire to redeem some good from embryos that have already been destroyed while not encouraging future embryo destruction. The present policy establishes three conditions:

- No federal funds have been or will be used in the destruction of embryos for research. There are 78 eligible cell lines, but no one is sure of their condition or how long these lines can remain viable.
- Those who use embryos destroyed after the date of the announcement will receive no federal funding.
- The president has reaffirmed the moral principle underlying his policy and the law on the subject.

In April 2004, 206 members of the House of Representatives signed a letter urging President Bush to modify his August 2001 executive order limiting the expenditure of federal funds to research using preexisting cell lines.

WHY IS FEDERAL FUNDING IMPORTANT?

Very strong emotions are present on both sides of the moral argument. The question is not whether research funds should be allowed for embryonic research, but whether the government should provide those funds. The American people have often provided support to scientific research that promises hope for human knowledge, health, and happiness. Some supporters argue that funding should extend ethical standards throughout all activities. Making public funds available allows the public scrutiny that will bring the critical review essential to ethical monitoring. When funding is entirely private, no one can be sure what the researchers are doing and what ethical standards may be broken.

The two sides appear to differ sharply on the basic moral significance of this question. One side believes research on human embryos is morally abhorrent in the extreme, while the other believes that such research is noble and even mandatory. Participants in this debate have addressed many complicated and difficult ethical matters, as presented in Chapter 10. The discussion centers on weighing and balancing the moral arguments, pondering the importance of relieving human suffering, giving researchers the freedom to conduct their research, and clarifying the moral standing of human embryos. To find common ground between the two positions, one must look at one's own moral beliefs and conscience.

In the United States a bill banning both therapeutic and reproductive cloning has passed in the House, but similar bills targeting therapeutic cloning have not passed in the Senate. Therapeutic cloning will probably never be banned because so many of the participants in the debate have relatives with diseases and disorders that are possible subjects of stem cell research. Several high-profile Republicans, including Senators Arlen Specter (R-PA), John McCain (R-AZ), and Orrin Hatch (R-UT) and former First Lady Nancy Reagan, are strongly supportive of stem cell research, although they do not necessarily agree that embryos should be made for the specific purpose of acquiring stem cells.

Current stem cell research policy can be summed up as follows:

1. President Bush is committed to enforcing the Dickey Amendment.
2. Even if there are scientific benefits, a majority of people in the Bush administration, in Congress, and among the public believe that taxpayer dollars should not be used to destroy human life.
3. Research on conquering disease is important but must respect moral boundaries.
4. Federal funding is important and should be awarded with care.

The current policy might appear to run helter-skelter in every direction. Federal funds are limited, but private researchers may continue to create lines from IVF embryos as long as their research is in compliance with state laws, which vary. In November 2004 California citizens approved Proposition 71 to issue bonds for $3 billion for ten years to fund stem cell research, including embryonic stem cell research. This places California in the position of spending more on the research than the rest of the world combined. In January 2005 New Jersey Governor James E. Greevey signed bill S1909, making New Jersey the second state to legalize stem cell research. Under this act, physicians treating patients for infertility are required to provide information allowing couples to make an informed and voluntary choice regarding the use of human embryos left over from IVF treatments. The act also prohibits human cloning. And on 6 April 2006 Maryland Governor Robert L. Ehrlich signed legislation to authorize $15 million for both adult and embryonic stem cell research for the coming year. Several other states, including Illinois, Massachusetts, Delaware, and Wisconsin, are considering initiatives for state-funded stem cell research to fill the federal funding gap.

Private funders are also stepping forward. Andrew Grove, founder of Intel Corp., will donate up to $5 million to the University of California at San Francisco for embryonic stem cell research, and the Michael J. Fox Foundation has given more than $5 million to institutions researching Parkinson's disease.

Federal funding of stem cell research continues to be a hot-button issue for candidates running for the U.S. House of Representatives and Senate. Understanding the official position of the United States is important to grasping the issues that are facing decision makers.

CHAPTER 12

Regulatory Issues in Other Countries

On 25 July 1978, the announcement of the birth of the first test-tube baby rocked the world. John and Lesley Brown, an English working-class couple, had tried for nine years to have a baby before Lesley was told that her damaged fallopian tubes blocked the passage of eggs. The Browns were referred to Dr. Patrick Steptoe, who had been collaborating with researcher Robert G. Edwards about a new procedure in which eggs (oocytes) were obtained from the mother and fertilized by the father's sperm outside the body. The fertilized embryo was then implanted in the uterus.

When baby Louise was born in the Oldham and General District Hospital in the north of England, it was also the birth of new hope for those who could not conceive. The Browns gave the little baby the middle name Joy because of their joy at being able to have this child. But after viewing a conceptus for the first time in newspapers, other possibilities were born in the minds of the public that day: the possibilities of manipulating embryos, and designing and cloning humans. The questions of ethics and the popular vision of the "brave new world" were again called into focus.

UNITED KINGDOM

Regulatory and legal issues first unfolded abroad, especially in the United Kingdom of England, Scotland, Northern Ireland, and Wales. Reacting to the practice of in vitro fertilization, the Human Fertilization and Embryology Authority was introduced in 1978 and was the subject of long and heated debates in the British parliament. Baroness Mary

Warnock was appointed chair of the Committee of Inquiry into Human Fertilization and Embryology, and the committee came out with a list of recommendations that were tabled in 1984. During that period, however, researchers with a volunteer license from an authority that oversaw infertility projects and IVF in the UK continued some investigations. After years of building trust among clinicians, researchers, and the public, parliament acted on the Human Fertilization and Embryology Act of 1990 (HFEA). HFEA basically implements the ideas of the committee and governs fertility and stem cell research in the United Kingdom.

The primitive streak that appears in the embryo around 14 days after fertilization marks the beginning of the formation of the central nervous system. The HFEA of 1990 prohibits research on embryos older than 14 days. Generally, a research license is granted only for the following reasons:

- To advance treatments for infertility
- To study causes of congenital diseases
- To increase knowledge about the causes of miscarriage
- To develop contraceptives
- To detect gene or chromosome abnormalities before implantation
- To promote other procedures that may advance medical treatments

When Dolly, the first cloned mammal, was born in 1996, a major concern about the possibility of human cloning led to passage of the Human Fertilization and Embryology Regulations (HFER). The act recommended that licenses for therapeutic cloning involving research on IVF embryos should require the 14-day limit. The concern that a surrogate mother might be used to bring a cloned human to full term led to passage of the Human Reproductive Cloning Act on 4 December 2001.

To deal with the issues of therapeutic cloning and stem cell research, the House of Lords called for hearings from a vast array of organizations representing many ethical positions. The committee reviewed the principles and focused on three elements:

1. The Abortion Act, which established an upper limit of 24 weeks for ending a pregnancy, was generally supported. It would not be logical to ban research on embryos when abortion was permitted past the time when the primitive streak was formed.
2. IVF in the UK had been practiced for more than 25 years and also had wide support. In that procedure, spare embryos are created that are later destroyed. It would be inconsistent to continue this practice and, at the same time, recognize that the embryo has legal status.

3. The 1990 HFEA with its provision of the 14-day rule had been enacted after much debate, and it had wide public support.

The committee agreed that embryos should not be created specifically for research unless there was an unusual need. Also, every cloned embryo must be accounted for, and research cannot extend beyond what the law allows.

EUROPEAN UNION

The European Union (EU) includes 14 countries on the continent of Europe, plus Ireland. The EU agrees with the UK about reproductive cloning and has passed laws to ban it. However, it disagrees on the issue of therapeutic cloning and passed Article 18 of the Council of Europe Convention on Human Rights and Biomedicine, a measure that prohibits the creation of embryos for research purposes. The EU contends that supporting abortion and prohibiting such research are two separate entities. Abortion has to do with the rights of the mother taking precedence over the rights of the fetus, but the rights of the embryos are paramount when abortion is not the issue. Any cloning that destroys human embryos is illegal in Germany, Austria, Poland, Portugal, Norway, and Ireland. Even the politically liberal Netherlands passed a ban on cloning. This group and the rest of the Council of Europe—40 countries, including Russia and Turkey—have banned therapeutic cloning.

Currently, the United Nations' 191 members unanimously support bans on cloning human babies, but they disagree on the issues of therapeutic cloning.

In addition to the United Kingdom, several countries (Singapore, China, Japan, Finland, Greece, Sweden, and Korea) permit culling stem cells from IVF embryos. Countries that have large Roman Catholic populations, such as Spain, France, Austria, Ireland, Germany, and Italy, oppose acquiring embryos from IVF or by cloning.

SINGAPORE

Singapore is a city-state that has rigid rules, and it expects its citizens to hold to high moral standards. It is a melting pot of Roman Catholics, Hindus, Buddhists, Bahaists, Taoists, Jews, and Sikhs. To sort out its citizens' feelings about harvesting stem cells from IVF embryos, the government appointed a bioethics committee representing each of the various religious groups and many professional groups to explore the positions and beliefs of each group about using stem cells in medicine. The government gave researchers free rein to use IVF embryos that had not grown past the thirteenth day, which allowed Ariff Bongso to develop several cell lines. The religious leaders searched their scriptures and their souls for answers to the question of religion and its relationship to science. The Roman Catholics and Sikhs did not agree, but the other religions accepted the practice of harvesting embryonic stem cells until the 14-day cutoff. Singapore is now a leader in providing IVF-derived stem cells.

ANATOMY OF A CONTROVERSY: SOUTH KOREA

South Korea has developed as a progressive nation in Asia and has become one of the major forces in stem cell research. It also excited a lot of discussion and questions when Woo Suk Hwang and colleagues at the Seoul National University announced in the journal *Science* on 12 February 2004 that they had cloned 30 human embryos and harvested stem cells from one of them. Headlines screamed that they were on the road to treating diseases such as Parkinson's. Other groups had claimed to have accomplished this feat also, but they did not have any supporting evidence. Biologists throughout the world alerted Western researchers that Asia was ahead of them and on the cutting edge. Hwang and colleagues told how they had collected 242 human eggs from 16 female volunteers, and they attributed their success to the supportive environment of their country, well-funded laboratories, and legislation that permitted the cloning of human embryos.

Investigators from the journal *Nature* questioned some of Hwang's ethical practices, because of the claim that some of the eggs might have come from junior members of his research team. Obtaining eggs is a risky and painful process and certainly is not a model for good practice. Hwang denied that what he was doing was wrong, but he agreed to suspend research until a new South Korean bioethics law came into effect the following year. At the annual meeting of the Korean Bioethics Association, members called on Hwang to answer questions about funding sources and the recruitment of egg donors. The association asked the National Human Rights Commission—an independent body—to investigate, but that task force was not intended to police specific research projects.

On 1 January 2005, the bioethics law came into effect and the government approved Hwang's embryonic stem cell research, the first approval issued under the new bioethics law. On 19 May 2005, Hwang's team made the news again with a report (*Science* 308, 1777–1783) of 11 embryonic stem cell lines derived from the skin cells of individual patients. It was hailed as a huge advance toward the medical use of stem cell research and also emphasized the embryo-cloning claims. In August 2005 came Snuppy, an Afghan hound that was the first dog to be cloned using the procedure. Some scientists questioned the value of dog cloning.

In October 2005, South Korea's government launched the World Stem Cell Hub, a huge international network for exchanging stem cell information and technology. Hwang, of course, was designated to head this worldwide network, which generated great interest from all over the world. According to BBC News (2005), more than 3,500 patients volunteered to take part in the research on the first day that applications were accepted. Contacts came by Internet, telephone, fax, and in person. Many who were victims of paralysis or other conditions were convinced that stem cell research was the answer.

In November, Gerald Schatten, a biologist at the University of Pittsburgh and one of Hwang's colleagues who co-authored the May 2005 *Science* paper, alleged that one of the researchers on the team—Sun Il Roh—had illegally traded ova. However, Schatten reassured *Science* that none of the eggs used in Hwang's two studies were obtained from reimbursed women donors. The paper's authors provided *Science* with corrections to data in a printed table that would greatly alter the conclusions, and Schatten publicly severed all ties to Hwang's team. Next, Sun Il Roh admitted that 20 eggs in the 2004 study were paid for but that Hwang did not know it.

On 22 November 2005, the Seoul-based Munhwa Broadcasting Corporation (MBC) issued an investigative report presenting additional evidence that Hwang used eggs from junior members of his lab. On 24 November he admitted that his stem cell research used eggs from paid donors and junior members of his team. He resigned from his official position but vowed to continue his research.

More trouble for Hwang developed when the MBC challenged the credibility of his studies' data. The program reported that the DNA in one of the cell lines did not match the tissue sample as it should. The mismatch raised the possibility that the embryonic stem cell lines were not cloned from the stated patients. On 4 December 2005, Hwang admitted to unintentional error in some of the data. Later that month, reports from collaborators alleged that the work was based on fabricated data and that possibly there were no cloned embryonic stem cells. Hwang apologized and admitted that there were some mistakes and human errors. The investigators at Seoul University delivered a condemning verdict: large amounts of the data in the papers were fabricated.

This controversy cast long shadows on stem cell research. It ignited old concerns about ethics, errors, and possible fraud. Claudia Dreifus (2006) interviewed Douglas Melton of the Harvard Stem Cell Center and asked if the Korean stem cell scandal surrounding Woo Suk Hwang's research made his work harder. Melton responded that it had raised the question in the public's mind of whether that kind of science had legitimacy. He added that even though Hwang's findings turned out to be fraudulent, nothing he claimed was a fundamental challenge to the principles of embryonic stem cell research. Melton said that the policies of the Bush administration had affected his research more significantly than Hwang's work, because many of America's brightest young scientists will not work in the stem cell area. Melton has private funding that allows his research to go on, but he must set up a whole new laboratory and have an accountant who makes sure that not a penny of federal funds goes to embryonic stem cell research. They must keep everything separate—computers, centrifuges, and even light bulbs.

Hwang had been considered a national hero in Korea, but the government revoked his license in the spring of 2006 and barred him from cloning or receiving human eggs for research.

Other countries, such as China and India, are reported to be interested in stem cell research, but currently do not have regulating bodies. Nations around the world vary in their approach to stem cell research. How the political winds will blow to cause a major shift in the paradigm is not predictable at this time.

CHAPTER 13

The Future of Stem Cell Research

If one observes the number of questions and problems surrounding stem cell research, it is almost like watching water flowing over Niagara Falls—mind-boggling. Some may yearn for the good old days when we knew little about embryos and thought less about them. The knowledge has crept up on us slowly. First there was in vitro fertilization, which posed the possibility of mixing eggs and sperm by the thousands in a petri dish. The results of fertilization could be sorted, graded, frozen, and even analyzed later for genetic defects. Later, scientists could take a five-day-old embryo, break it open, spread out the cells, and develop embryonic cell lines. Those broken embryos caused some people to question the morality of the process. Was it cold-blooded murder of an embryo to fulfill some vision that people might have of curing certain diseases? Both sides of the issue began to present their points of view—loudly. Now it is like the roar of Niagara.

Misunderstanding and misconception also rear their ugly heads. In the course of their science education, students are taught very little about the basic molecular biology of the process, and therefore they have little foundation as adults to understand the plethora of new discoveries and technology in stem cell research. Thus they become like the Delta group of *Brave New World*—easy to lead and manipulate. The public expects things to be explained in simple, 30-second sound bites, but it probably takes an hour or more to develop the background for even a basic understanding of this complex subject. When television specials do try to explain the process and issues, hoping to improve their ratings, they promote the program with sensational titles such as "Making Perfect People." Slogans and the usual mass media messages cannot work with the complicated subject of stem cells. Stars and celebrities such as Christopher Reeve, Mary Tyler Moore, and Michael J. Fox have brought the subject of stem cell research to the attention of the public, but generally they have not explained in detail what the process involves.

Despite the ethical and moral questions, high costs and risks, and huge regulatory hurdles, research into the therapeutic potential of stem cells continues. For those who support the research, it is the fair-haired child that brings promise of cures for debilitating diseases. Those who oppose the research claim it is the wicked witch and the black sheep that promise only doom to the humanity of the race.

Apparently, the general public supports stem cell research. According to a 2004 Harris Poll that asked if stem cell research should be allowed, a 6-to-1 majority favored the research. That result reflected an increase compared with poll results in 2001, when the majority favored research by only 3 to 1 (Ribbink, 2005). But a major problem that appears when looking at this poll question is that it was not specific as to the type of stem cell research. Some people may support adult stem cell research but oppose embryonic research.

The spending of money for stem cell research is apparently not slackening. According to the NIH, about $230 million was spent on all human stem cell research in 2004. Wise Young, MD, PhD, of Rutgers University thinks this is a paltry amount, considering the benefits that stem cell research could provide (Ribbink, 2005). According to Navigant Consulting, Inc. (2005), money is being spent, and as public funding increases, private funding will also increase. The total amount of public funding for stem cell research in the United States, about $230 million in 2004, tripled to about $630 million in 2005. Two leading companies—California-based Geron Corporation and ES Cells—will benefit from California's favorable funding referendum. Navigant analysts predict that the first stem cell therapeutics will be commercialized in the United States by 2009; ViaCell Inc.'s adult stem cell–based cancer treatment, derived from cord blood, will be the first product to market. By 2015, treatments for diabetes and cardiovascular disorders will lead the way as the U.S. stem cell market reaches more than $3.6 billion in revenues. See Table 13.1, Stem Cell Market Share by Therapeutic Area (2015). Adult stem cell therapies will lead the way in market growth initially, but embryonic therapeutics will overtake that market by 2012.

However, critics see the billions of dollars spent on stem cell research as one of the signs that this black sheep is leading us to impending doom. In a 2006 opinion piece, Charles Colson comments on how the South Korean government had revoked the license of Woo Suk Hwang and had admitted that he was a notorious con man. He questions the supporters of

Table 13.1   Stem Cell Market Share by Therapeutic Area (2015)

Condition	Percentage
Diabetes	48
Cardiovascular	27
Spinal cord regeneration	7
Reconstruction of blood system	5
HIV	4
Bone regeneration	4
GVHD	3
Chondrocyte	2
Others	<1

Source: Evelyn B. Kelly, from information in Ribbink (2005).

embryonic stem cell research who claim that Hwang's debacle was an individual problem and not a problem of scientific inquiry. Also, Colson contends that the tremendous money spent on stem cell research is strictly business, an effort to obtain patents and make even more money. The dishonesty that abounds in embryonic stem cell research helps secure patents, not cure patients. It is far more lucrative than research involving adult stem cells, and Colson advises his readers to follow the money. He claims that scientific venture capital will be used to form biotech companies that develop patents to sell to biotech or pharmaceutical firms, and that these industries do not really want to develop scientific cures.

Opinions about stem cell research continue to come from many directions. Some scientists are convinced that if we can work together to really understand this complex topic, a consensus will develop to move research forward in a safe manner. Robert P. Kelch, the University of Michigan's executive vice president for medical affairs, respects diverse positions and does not disagree that a blastocyst has the potential for human life. In an interview with Sally Pobojewski (2005), Kelch advocated some resolution of the problem of 300,000 to 400,000 frozen blastocysts (early embryos) that have been created for in vitro fertilization. Many of these embryos are going to be discarded, but they have tremendous potential to be used for the greater good.

Kelch believes in putting a lot of money into cancer stem cells, cord blood stem cells, and adult or tissue cells because we are going to learn a lot from them, but the fact remains that embryonic stem cells have the amazing potential to give rise to all of the tissues in the entire body. Nevertheless, he believes that there are certain things that should remain off-limits to scientists. Doing certain things in humans that might be acceptable in animal studies is unethical. Making chimeras or mixing different genetic cell lines to develop chimeras is unethical in relation to human beings. Working on human embryos that are beyond the implantation stage is unethical.

Scientists agree that stem cell science is in its infancy. Intensive basic science research is necessary before any safety test, regulatory approval, or product commercialization can occur.

BANKING ON STEM CELLS

Chapter 4 looked at the process of growing and maintaining stem cells and discussed the possible use of cord blood. Since the 1980s, private and public cord banks have vied for umbilical cord blood, which is used to treat leukemia, lymphoma, aplastic anemia, sickle cell anemia, and other immune and genetic disorders. When South Korea announced the opening of an embryonic stem cell bank in the spring of 2005, the U.S. government was poised to open a stem cell bank of a different kind—a public bank for cord blood–derived stem cells.

Steven Reinberg (2005) reports that transplantation from cord blood cells has saved the lives of about 200,000 people, and each year some 1,700 patients get a stem cell transplant. However, estimates suggest that about 11,700 people could benefit from these cells each year. There are about 40 public banks in the world, including 20 in the United States. An additional 15 for-profit banks store blood for a fee. Reinberg quotes from an Institute of Medicine (IOM) report issued in April 2005 that as part of the Stem Cell Therapeutic and Research Act of 2005, the United States will set aside $79 million in funding over the next five years. The Senate and House are considering bills that will set aside a portion of those dollars for organizing public cord blood banking and establishing new standards. The current system has a number of problems, including a lack of standards for collecting and storing blood, an inability to match patients and donors in a rapid and efficient manner, and an insufficient number of stored units. The median time for locating an HLA match is about four months, according to the IOM report, and increasing the number of banks will increase the possibility of finding a match.

FUTURISTIC SOURCES

In the forefront, the search is on to find a practical source for stem cells that everyone can support. Adult stem cells from a variety of sources such as bone marrow, umbilical cord blood, amniotic fluid, body fat, skin, baby teeth, and cadavers have been the subject of prominent press releases. Finding a noncontroversial source would be a great boon for stem cell research, but the question remains, will new ways of creating stem cells dodge the objections? Many proposals and ideas are floating around that hope to answer this question. Here are some of the proposals.

Cloning—But Not Really

This proposal is cloning with a twist. The scientist would genetically manipulate the nucleus of a somatic (body) cell before transferring it into an egg whose nucleus has been removed. One or more of the genes necessary for orderly development would be inactivated. All types of tissue then could form in a haphazard and unorganized way, but would not create a new human being. Proponents of this technique argue that no embryo exists because the developmental parts are missing, so it is not unethical to take it apart to make stem cells.

This idea is not new, although the President's Council for Bioethics just recently took up the question. ACT, a biotechnology company, applied for a patent on the technique in 2002. However, some still contend that the process is an abuse of cloning technology and that a short-lived embryo is still an embryo.

A Nonviable Embryo

A second proposal before the Council on Bioethics is to have scientists determine that an embryo is not viable and then use the cells from that embryo. This argument is like the analogy of brain death and organ transplantations, where tissues are removed from newly dead cadavers. The question is how to determine when an embryo is not viable.

Human Cells in Nonhuman Eggs

To study targeted diseases at the cellular level, human somatic cells may be transferred into nonhuman eggs to produce nuclear transferred-human embryonic stem cell (NT-hESC) lines. These cells are not targeted for transplant, but are used to study diseases and disorders. For example, Ian Wilmut of the Roslin Institute in Edinburgh, Scotland, announced in 2006 plans to use rabbit eggs for NT-hESC research to examine the progression of human motor neuron diseases.

Fusing Adult and Embryonic Cells

Research on the fusion of adult and embryonic cells is in the early stages of development at the Harvard Stem Cell Institute. Scientists have created cells that are similar to stem cells by fusing human skin cells with embryonic stem cells. The result is a hybrid that looks and acts like stem cells. The implication here is that it may be possible to create tailor-made, genetically matched stem cells using cell fusion, rather than by destroying early embryos. Gareth Cook and Carey Goldberg (2005) reported that Kevin Egan and colleagues published the results of their fusion research in August 2005 in the journal *Science*. However, Egan emphasized that fusion research is not yet "ready for prime time" and is still inefficient at this point.

The work is part of a broader effort to conduct embryonic research without destroying embryos. The procedure would allow scientists to create a vast number of embryonic stem cells, thereby enabling experimentation to determine what happens when an adult cell is transformed into an embryonic stem cell—a process called **reprogramming.** It has long been a dream of scientists to make an adult cell regress to the embryonic stem cell state without involving an egg cell. The fusion process differs from cloning, which uses an egg cell and involves putting the nucleus from a skin cell into the nucleus of the egg.

A couple of obstacles remain, however. First, the new cells contain twice the genetic material that cells normally carry, and at present there is no way to reduce the amount of genetic information. One answer is to pull out the extra DNA before the fusion process is complete. Another option might be to reprogram the skin cells using the stem cell's cytoplasm, the area outside the nucleus that contains DNA. Harvard scientists are designing experiments to help resolve the problems of fusion.

A second obstacle is the inefficiency of the process. Scientists creating the fused cells found that 50 million embryonic stem cells and 50 million skin cells yielded only 10 to 20 of the hybrid fused cells, although the fused cells were stable. Such cells would be risky for therapy, although they could be useful for research.

Regeneration: Growing One's Own Stem Cells

Chapter 2 discusses the history of scientists who were fascinated by the regeneration of body parts in some animals. Rene-Antoine Ferchault de Reaumur was probably the first to observe regeneration, and he presented his study to the French Academy in 1712. Later, Abraham Trembly found that the hydra, a small water animal, could regenerate body parts, just as the mythological Hydra did. Early investigators never pondered why regeneration occurred, and later it was found that some mammals also regenerate parts of the body. Deer, for example, can regrow antlers at the rate of about two centimeters per day. The liver of a mammal is a startling example of regeneration. Scientists speculate that the liver can regenerate in two to three weeks, even if 75 percent of the organ is damaged during surgery. This ability may be a response to bad food, plant toxins, and viruses that have exposed the liver to damage throughout the evolutionary process.

If the tip of the finger is severed above the last joint, it will sometimes regenerate. Why does this happen? Regeneration begins when mature cells at the site of the wound revert to an immature state, called a blastema. The blastema appears to get its instructions from cells at the wound site, so the machinery must be part of the genetic equipment. But for some reason, the genes have fallen into disuse. Nicholas Wade (2006) reported that Dr. Mark Keating of Novartis (Cambridge, MA), identified a gene that initiates the formation of a blastema in zebra fish. The same kind of gene, fgf20, and another kind, hsp60, also exist in humans, which suggests that a genetic mechanism may be in place.

One of the few laboratories in the world that is investigating regeneration is at the University of Utah. Shannon Odelberg is studying regeneration in the newt, with the hope of finding ways to induce blastema formation in mammals.

Some scientists who support regeneration believe stem cell therapy may not be as close to reality as the advocates sometimes suggest. Stem cell theory does not agree with the principles of the blastema mechanism. The blastema's reliance on internal information from the cell contrasts with a principal assumption of stem cell therapy: that stem cells inserted into damaged tissue will use local cues to integrate into the surrounding tissue. Supporters of the stem cell position point to bone marrow transplantation as the big story on which much of the hope for stem cell therapy is based. The reality is that both regeneration and stem cell therapy are still in their infancy, and decades will pass before either of the two procedures will prove itself.

Parthenotes

Parthenotes are unfertilized eggs that are stimulated by chemical or electrical impulses and grown to the blastocyst state, so the stem cells can be harvested. Certain species of insects, frogs, fish, and lizards reproduce by parthenogenesis, in which an egg develops without a sperm. In April 2004, researchers developed a mouse parthenote. This parthenote cannot go into the fetal stage because it lacks the paternal DNA that promotes development of the umbilical cord. Some scientists reason that because it is not an embryo, a parthenote could provide stem cells that would not be controversial. But no one knows if those stem cell lines would be scientifically or clinically useful. Critics say that the more parthenotes are believed to function like embryos, the more objectionable they become.

Pre-implantation Genetic Diagnosis (PGD)

Currently, a few cells can be taken from a healthy embryo to determine if certain genetic defects or disorders are present, and some researchers suggest that such cells could be used to make stem cell lines. However, others are not sure that these cells would form viable stem cell lines, and the ethical problem of experimentation would still exist. Although healthy children have been born after PGD, it is still a risky and uncertain procedure, because no one knows what will happen after some cells are split off from the embryo. Is it morally appropriate to risk damage to a healthy embryo?

FUTURE ETHICAL ISSUES

Korean folklore tells the story of the nation's origin. Pak Hyeokkeise was the first ruler of Shiila, the ancient Buddhist state that became Korea. Six rulers of the land prayed for a king who would lead Shiila, and gathered to pray for guidance. A sudden flash of lightning revealed a giant egg, and from the egg stepped the young boy who would be their king. This metaphor for the origin of the country is like the hope that South Koreans saw in Dr. Woo Suk Hwang at Seoul University, only this time the magical Korean egg was created through somatic cell nuclear transfer. And like a mythical story, Hwang's scientific papers turned out to be fiction. On 10 January 2006, the investigating committee issued its final report and revoked the researcher's license.

After the initial shock of scandal among the ranks, scientists in other countries have forged ahead to take the lead in nuclear transferred-human embryonic stem cell (NT-hESC) research, or cloning. Research has accelerated at the Harvard Stem Cell Institute, Advanced Cell Technology, the University of California (San Francisco), the University of California (Los Angeles), Karolinska Institute in Sweden, Newcastle University (UK), Queen's Medical Research Institute at the University of Edinburgh, and the Institute of Psychiatry in London. Rather than discouraging research, the South Korean scandal appears to have had the very opposite effect of encouraging it.

However, these new research opportunities are faced with the same threats of danger that plagued the South Korean researchers. The National Academies' National Research Council and the Institute of Medicine (2005) issued a joint report establishing standards for embryonic stem cell research that included deriving, storing, distributing, and using embryonic stem cell lines. The guidelines call for Embryonic Stem Cell Research Oversight (ESCRO) committees to review protocols and maintain registries of lines banked at their institutions.

Insoo Hyun of the Hastings Institute (2006) has suggested that although the ethics of egg donation have received considerable attention, three other ethical issues also must be considered:

- While concentrating on human egg donation, scientists have ignored the ethics of somatic cell donation, an element that may outlast the question about eggs. For example, if artificial eggs are created from embryonic stem cells by one of the futuristic procedures listed earlier in this chapter, the somatic cell from a human must still be used.
- People who are participating in the research must understand what they are doing when they donate somatic cells. Subjects must not have the therapeutic misconception that every aspect of the research project was designed to benefit them directly. They must understand what the terms *random sample* and *double-blind* mean in scientific research.
- Research to enhance the informed consent procedures for donating both eggs and somatic cells is a dire need. Understanding the interests of donors, their misconceptions, and what they know about the informed consent process is essential. Research conducted among minorities and in other countries must reflect their cultural understanding of informed consent.

POWERFUL ADVOCATES

Both sides of the stem cell controversy have powerful advocates. Chapter 10 considered the positions of various religious leaders and objections from conservatives and Roman Catholics that are built primarily around the moral status of the embryo.

Other advocates focus on the end as being great enough to justify the means. Mary Tyler Moore (2006), the television celebrity, is one of those advocates. Moore has lived with type 1 (juvenile) diabetes for 35 years. She has described how this personal time bomb has threatened her through much of her life. Using many case histories, Moore and Michael J. Fox, a victim of Parkinson's disease, testified before Congress in support of funding for stem cell research. They especially focused on the thousands of eggs that would become the discards of in vitro fertilization. Christopher Reeve (2006) stated that when he became a patient advocate in 1995, he thought funding would be the major problem. Instead, he found that the main obstacles involved embryonic stem cell research and therapeutic cloning. Reeve concluded that the first task would be to dispel misinformation. Advocates point out how moral and ethical questions have always dogged new ideas, but they encourage the United States to change its policy before it falls behind other countries that are progressing in stem cell research.

EDUCATION MUST RESPOND

Students must learn not only about basic biology but also about the processes that are taking place in the fields of genetics and cell biology relating to stem cells. The subject of embryology in general science textbooks is almost nonexistent, or weak at best. High school biology courses seldom mention stem cell research, possibly because teachers have little background in it themselves. These conditions must change in order to create an educated public that can support and make decisions. Educators concerned about no child being left behind must make certain that their wards are not left behind in obtaining a foundation for understanding scientific advances.

Only with wisdom and understanding of the issues, and by being able to articulate a position, can our society benefit from technology yet preserve our humanity.

SECTION THREE

References and Resources

Section One, consisting of Chapters 1 through 7, presents the foundations of the science that established stem cell research. Section One considers the historical development and scientific background of stem cell research, the growth and maintenance of embryonic stem cells, and the diseases and disorders targeted for research. Section Two, consisting of Chapters 8 through 13, considers ethical, religious, and regulatory issues. This section provides the reader with references and resources consisting of primary documents that established the foundations of ethical and policy decisions. A brief of *Roe v. Wade* is given, along with the majority opinion written by Justic Blackmun and the dissenting opinion written by Justice Rehnquist.

Annotated Primary Source Documents

OATH WRITTEN BY HIPPOCRATES, CA. 400 BC

Chapter 9 addressed ethics and research in history. The word "ethics" comes from the Greek *ethos,* meaning character. No document embodies the ethics of the medical profession better than the oath accredited to Hippocrates of Cos, written around 400 BC. Hippocrates lived at a time when treatment of the sick involved superstition and incantations. Sometimes very poisonous and dangerous methods were used. Hippocrates disagreed with that approach and sought to develop a kinder and gentler way of treating people. He was convinced that no treatment should be harsh or inhumane.

Later, followers of Hippocrates redefined the medical profession in terms of the Hippocratic Oath. During the Dark Ages (medieval period) the oath was forgotten, but it was revived during the Renaissance and published around 1525. Today, graduates of medical schools take the Hippocratic Oath as they begin their practice of medicine. Francis Adams translated this version.

The Oath of Hippocrates

I SWEAR by Apollo the physician, and Aesculapius, and Health, and All-heal, and all the gods and goddesses, that, according to my ability and judgment, I will keep this Oath and this stipulation—to reckon him who taught me this Art equally dear to me as my parents, to share my substance with him, and relieve his necessities if required; to look upon his offspring in the same footing as my own brothers, and to teach them this art, if they shall wish to learn it, without fee or stipulation; and that by precept, lecture, and every other mode of instruction, I will impart a knowledge of the Art to my own sons, and those of my teachers, and to disciples bound by a stipulation and oath according to the law of medicine, but to none others. I will follow that system of regimen which, according to my ability and judgment, I consider for the benefit of my patients, and abstain from whatever is deleterious and mischievous. I will give no deadly medicine to any one if asked, nor suggest any such counsel; and in like manner I will not give to a woman a pessary to produce abortion. With purity and with holiness I will pass my life and practice my Art. I will not cut persons laboring under the stone, but will leave this to be done by men who are practitioners of this work. Into whatever houses I enter, I will go into them for the benefit of the sick, and will abstain from every voluntary act of mischief and corruption; and, further from the seduction of females or males, of freemen and slaves. Whatever, in connection with my professional practice or not, in connection with it, I see or hear, in the life of men, which ought not to be spoken of abroad, I will not divulge, as reckoning that all such should be kept secret. While I continue to keep this Oath unviolated, may it be granted to me to enjoy life and the practice of the art, respected by all men, in all times! But should I trespass and violate this Oath, may the reverse be my lot!

THE BERLIN CODE OF 1900

As scientific information expanded at the end of the nineteenth century, many investigators began to ponder ethical questions about certain experiments with humans. Rudolf Virchow, a microbiologist in Berlin, had serious reservations about some of the trials being done in the name of science. When Neisser found the spirochete organism that he believed to cause syphilis, he inoculated some unsuspecting subjects with serum from patients with the disease. Virchow was outraged by such lack of concern for human beings, and he convinced the Berlin City Council to write a code of conduct.

That code was one of the first and strongest codes to specify ethical conditions for medical research, but it was short-lived. In 1931 Adolph Hitler signed a memo stating that the code did not apply to Jews, Gypsies, people with mental disabilities, and others. He said that they were not citizens and were not entitled to the code's protection. Nevertheless, the Berlin Code is an important historical document that made a powerful statement. It can be found on the Internet at http://www.geocities.com/artandersonmd/00prussion1900.jpg.

The Royal Prussian Minister of Religious, Educational and Medical Affairs
   Directive to all medical directors of university hospitals, polyclinics,
    and other hospitals

 I. I advise the medical directors of university hospitals, polyclinics, and all other hospitals that all medical interventions for othter than diagnostic, healing, and immunization purposes, regardless of other legal or moral authorization, are excluded under all circumstances, if
  (1) the human subject is a minor or not competent due to other reasons;
  (2) the human subject has not given his unambiguous consent;

(3) the consent is not preceded by a proper explanation of the possible negative consequences of the intervention.

II.   At the same time I determine that
(1) interventions of this kind are to be only performed by the medical director himself or with his special authorization;
(2) in all cases of these interventions the fulfillment of the requirements of I (1–3) and II (1), as well as all further circumstances of the case, are documented in the medical record.

III.   The existing instructions about medical interventions for diagnostic, healing, and immunization purposes are not affected by these instructions.

Berlin, 29 December 1900
The Minister for Religious ec. Affairs
Studt

THE NUREMBERG CODE

The Nuremberg Code resulted from the trials of Nazi criminals at Nuremberg, Germany, in 1946, after World War II. In the name of scientific progress, Nazi doctors had performed horrible experiments on prisoners at the concentration camps. This code was developed to establish a foundation for the ethical treatment of people—first to do no harm, but then to ensure voluntary consent. People who engage in medical trials today must sign a form saying that they voluntarily give their consent for treatment and that they understand what will happen to them in terms of risks, duration of the experiment, and other important details.

Text of the Nuremberg Code

The Nuremberg Military Tribunal's decision in the case of the *United States v. Karl Brandt et al.* includes what is now called the Nuremberg Code, a ten-point statement delimiting permissible medical experimentation on human subjects. According to this statement, human experimentation is justified only if its results benefit society and it is carried out in accord with basic principles that "satisfy moral, ethical, and legal concepts." To some extent, the Nuremberg Code has been superseded by the Declaration of Helsinki as a guide for human experimentation because The Code does not address Clinical Research in Patients with Illnesses

1.   The voluntary consent of the human subject is absolutely essential.

This means that the person involved should have legal capacity to give consent; should be so situated as to be able to exercise free power of choice, without the intervention of any element of force, fraud, deceit, duress, over-reaching, or other ulterior form of constraint or coercion; and should have sufficient knowledge and comprehension of the elements of the subject matter involved as to enable him to make an understanding and enlightened decision. This latter element requires that before the acceptance of an affirmative decision by the experimental subject there should be made known to him the nature, duration, and purpose of the experiment; the method and means by which it is to be conducted; all inconveniences and hazards reasonably to be expected; and the effects upon his health or person which may possibly come from his participation in the experiment.

The duty and responsibility for ascertaining the quality of the consent rests upon each individual who initiates, directs or engages in the experiment. It is a personal duty and responsibility which may not be delegated to another with impunity.

2. **The experiment should be such as to yield fruitful results for the good of society, unprocurable by other methods or means of study, and not random and unnecessary in nature.**

3. **The experiment should be so designed and based on the results of animal experimentation and a knowledge of the natural history of the disease or other problem under study that the anticipated results will justify the performance of the experiment.**

4. **The experiment should be so conducted as to avoid all unnecessary physical and mental suffering and injury.**

5. **No experiment should be conducted where there is an a priori reason to believe that death or disabling injury will occur; "except, perhaps, in those experiments where the experimental physicians also serve as subjects."**

6. **The degree of risk to be taken should never exceed that determined by the humanitarian importance of the problem to be solved by the experiment.**

7. **Proper preparations should be made and adequate facilities provided to protect the experimental subject against even remote possibilities of injury, disability, or death.**

8. **The experiment should be conducted only by scientifically qualified persons. The highest degree of skill and care should be required through all stages of the experiment of those who conduct or engage in the experiment.**

9. **During the course of the experiment the human subject should be at liberty to bring the experiment to an end if he has reached the physical or mental state where continuation of the experiment seems to him to be impossible.**

10. **During the course of the experiment the scientist in charge must be prepared to terminate the experiment at any stage, if he has probable cause to believe, in the exercise of the good faith, superior skill and careful judgment required of him that a continuation of the experiment is likely to result in injury, disability, or death to the experimental subject.**

Source: "Permissible Medical Experiments." *Trials of War Criminals before the Nuremberg Military Tribunals under Control Council Law No. 10: Nuremberg October 1946–April 1949.* Washington, DC: U.S. Government Printing Office (n.d.), vol. 2, pp. 181–182.

Quotes were added around the self-experimentation clause of item 5 because it would be irresponsible for the person whose knowledge was essential for the safety and welfare of subjects to render himself incapacitated by taking the test agent along with his subjects.

THE BELMONT REPORT

When the U.S. Public Health Service revealed that a study of syphilis in Tuskegee, Alabama, had been sanctioned from 1932 to 1972, the world was shocked. The fact that the service withheld known treatment that could have cured the men was indeed a low point for medical experimentation. The Tuskegee revelations led to the National Research Act (PL 93-348) in July 1974, which added additional restrictions and oversight to research involving human subjects. On 12 July 1975, a commission was formed to identify basic ethical principles that should govern any research involving human subjects. The name of the following report comes from the Belmont Conference Center at the Smithsonian Institution.

The Belmont Report

Ethical Principles and Guidelines for the Protection of Human Subjects of Research

---

The National Commission for the Protection of Human Subjects of Biomedical and Behavioral Research

April 18, 1979

AGENCY: Department of Health, Education, and Welfare

ACTION: Notice of Report for Public Comment

SUMMARY: On July 12, 1974, the National Research Act (Pub. L. 93-348) was signed into law, thereby creating the National Commission for the Protection of

Human Subjects of Biomedical and Behavioral Research. One of the charges to the Commission was to identify the basic ethical principles that should underlie the conduct of biomedical and behavioral research involving human subjects and to develop guidelines which should be followed to assure that such research is conducted in accordance with those principles. In carrying out the above, the Commission was directed to consider: (i) the boundaries between biomedical and behavioral research and the accepted and routine practice of medicine, (ii) the role of assessment of risk-benefit criteria in the determination of the appropriateness of research involving human subjects, (iii) appropriate guidelines for the selection of human subjects for participation in such research and (iv) the nature and definition of informed consent in various research settings.

The Belmont Report attempts to summarize the basic ethical principles identified by the Commission in the course of its deliberations. It is the outgrowth of an intensive four-day period of discussions that were held in February 1976 at the Smithsonian Institution's Belmont Conference Center supplemented by the monthly deliberations of the Commission that were held over a period of nearly four years. It is a statement of basic ethical principles and guidelines that should assist in resolving the ethical problems that surround the conduct of research with human subjects. By publishing the Report in the Federal Register, and providing reprints upon request, the Secretary intends that it may be made readily available to scientists, members of Institutional Review Boards, and Federal employees. The two-volume Appendix, containing the lengthy reports of experts and specialists who assisted the Commission in fulfilling this part of its charge, is available as DHEW Publication No. (OS) 78-0013 and No. (OS) 78-0014, for sale by the Superintendent of Documents, U.S. Government Printing Office, Washington, D.C. 20402.

Unlike most other reports of the Commission, the Belmont Report does not make specific recommendations for administrative action by the Secretary of Health, Education, and Welfare. Rather, the Commission recommended that the Belmont Report be adopted in its entirety, as a statement of the Department's policy. The Department requests public comment on this recommendation.

National Commission for the Protection of Human Subjects of Biomedical and Behavioral Research

Members of the Commission

Kenneth John Ryan, M.D., Chairman, Chief of Staff, Boston Hospital for Women

Joseph V. Brady, Ph.D., Professor of Behavioral Biology, Johns Hopkins University

Robert E. Cooke, M.D., President, Medical College of Pennsylvania

Dorothy I. Height, President, National Council of Negro Women, Inc.

Albert R. Jonsen, Ph.D., Associate Professor of Bioethics, University of California at San Francisco

Patricia King, J.D., Associate Professor of Law, Georgetown University Law Center

Karen Lebacqz, Ph.D., Associate Professor of Christian Ethics, Pacific School of Religion

* David W. Louisell, J.D., Professor of Law, University of California at Berkeley

Donald W. Seldin, M.D., Professor and Chairman, Department of Internal Medicine, University of Texas at Dallas

Eliot Stellar, Ph.D., Provost of the University and Professor of Physiological Psychology, University of Pennsylvania

* Robert H. Turtle, LL.B., Attorney, VomBaur, Coburn, Simmons & Turtle, Washington, D.C.

* Deceased

Ethical Principles and Guidelines for Research Involving Human Subjects

Scientific research has produced substantial social benefits. It has also posed some troubling ethical questions. Public attention was drawn to these questions by reported abuses of human subjects in biomedical experiments, especially during the Second World War. During the Nuremberg War Crime Trials, the Nuremberg Code was drafted as a set of standards for judging physicians and scientists who had conducted biomedical experiments on concentration camp prisoners. This code became the prototype of many later codes[1] intended to assure that research involving human subjects would be carried out in an ethical manner.

The codes consist of rules, some general, others specific, that guide the investigators or the reviewers of research in their work. Such rules often are inadequate to cover complex situations; at times they come into conflict, and they are frequently difficult to interpret or apply. Broader ethical principles will provide a basis on which specific rules may be formulated, criticized and interpreted.

Three principles, or general prescriptive judgments, that are relevant to research involving human subjects are identified in this statement. Other principles may also be relevant. These three are comprehensive, however, and are stated at a level of generalization that should assist scientists, subjects, reviewers and interested citizens to understand the ethical issues inherent in research involving human subjects. These principles cannot always be applied so as to resolve beyond dispute particular ethical problems. The objective is to provide an analytical framework that will guide the resolution of ethical problems arising from research involving human subjects.

This statement consists of a distinction between research and practice, a discussion of the three basic ethical principles, and remarks about the application of these principles.

Part A: Boundaries Between Practice & Research

It is important to distinguish between biomedical and behavioral research, on the one hand, and the practice of accepted therapy on the other, in order to know what activities ought to undergo review for the protection of human subjects of research. The distinction between research and practice is blurred partly because both often occur together (as in research designed to evaluate a therapy) and partly because notable departures from standard practice are often called "experimental" when the terms "experimental" and "research" are not carefully defined.

For the most part, the term "practice" refers to interventions that are designed solely to enhance the well-being of an individual patient or client and that have a reasonable expectation of success. The purpose of medical or behavioral practice is to provide diagnosis, preventive treatment or therapy to particular individuals.[2] By contrast, the term "research" designates an activity designed to test an hypothesis, permit conclusions to be drawn, and thereby to develop or contribute to generalizable knowledge (expressed, for example, in theories, principles, and statements of relationships). Research is usually described in a formal protocol that sets forth an objective and a set of procedures designed to reach that objective.

When a clinician departs in a significant way from standard or accepted practice, the innovation does not, in and of itself, constitute research. The fact that a procedure is "experimental," in the sense of new, untested or different, does not automatically place it in the category of research. Radically new procedures of this description should, however, be made the object of formal research at an early stage in order to determine whether they are safe and effective. Thus, it is the responsibility of medical practice committees, for example, to insist that a major innovation be incorporated into a formal research project.[3]

Research and practice may be carried on together when research is designed to evaluate the safety and efficacy of a therapy. This need not cause any confusion regarding whether or not the activity requires review; the general rule is that if there is any element of research in an activity, that activity should undergo review for the protection of human subjects.

Part B: Basic Ethical Principles

The expression "basic ethical principles" refers to those general judgments that serve as a basic justification for the many particular ethical prescriptions and evaluations of human actions. Three basic principles, among those generally accepted in our cultural tradition, are particularly relevant to the ethics of research involving human subjects: the principles of respect for persons, beneficence and justice.

1. Respect for Persons—Respect for persons incorporates at least two ethical convictions: first, that individuals should be treated as autonomous agents, and second, that persons with diminished autonomy are entitled to protection. The principle of respect for persons thus divides into two separate moral requirements: the requirement to acknowledge autonomy and the requirement to protect those with diminished autonomy.

An autonomous person is an individual capable of deliberation about personal goals and of acting under the direction of such deliberation. To respect autonomy is to give weight to autonomous persons' considered opinions and choices while refraining from obstructing their actions unless they are clearly detrimental to others. To show lack of respect for an autonomous agent is to repudiate that person's considered judgments, to deny an individual the freedom to act on those considered judgments, or to withhold information necessary to make a considered judgment, when there are no compelling reasons to do so.

However, not every human being is capable of self-determination. The capacity for self-determination matures during an individual's life, and some individuals lose this capacity wholly or in part because of illness, mental disability, or circumstances that severely restrict liberty. Respect for the immature and the incapacitated may require protecting them as they mature or while they are incapacitated.

Some persons are in need of extensive protection, even to the point of excluding them from activities which may harm them; other persons require little protection beyond making sure they undertake activities freely and with awareness of possible adverse consequence. The extent of protection afforded should depend upon the risk of harm and the likelihood of benefit. The judgment that any individual lacks autonomy should be periodically reevaluated and will vary in different situations.

In most cases of research involving human subjects, respect for persons demands that subjects enter into the research voluntarily and with adequate information. In some situations, however, application of the principle is not obvious. The involvement of prisoners as subjects of research provides an instructive example. On the one hand, it would seem that the principle of respect for persons requires that prisoners not be deprived of the opportunity to volunteer for research. On the other hand, under prison conditions they may be subtly coerced or unduly influenced to engage in research activities for which they would not otherwise volunteer. Respect for persons would then dictate that prisoners be protected. Whether to allow prisoners to "volunteer" or to "protect" them presents a dilemma. Respecting persons, in most hard cases, is often a matter of balancing competing claims urged by the principle of respect itself.

2. Beneficence—Persons are treated in an ethical manner not only by respecting their decisions and protecting them from harm, but also by making efforts to secure their well-being. Such treatment falls under the principle of beneficence. The term "beneficence" is often understood to cover acts of kindness or charity that go beyond strict obligation. In this document, beneficence is understood in a stronger sense, as an obligation. Two general rules have been formulated as complementary expressions of beneficent actions in this sense: (1) do not harm and (2) maximize possible benefits and minimize possible harms.

The Hippocratic maxim "do no harm" has long been a fundamental principle of medical ethics. Claude Bernard extended it to the realm of research, saying that one should not injure one person regardless of the benefits that might come to others. However, even avoiding harm requires learning what is harmful; and, in the process of obtaining this information, persons may be exposed to risk of harm. Further, the Hippocratic Oath requires physicians to benefit their patients "according to their best judgment." Learning what will in fact benefit may require exposing persons to risk. The problem posed by these imperatives is to decide when it is justifiable to seek certain benefits despite the risks involved, and when the benefits should be foregone because of the risks.

The obligations of beneficence affect both individual investigators and society at large, because they extend both to particular research projects and to the entire enterprise of research. In the case of particular projects, investigators and members of their institutions are obliged to give forethought to the maximization of benefits and the reduction of risk that might occur from the research investigation. In the case of scientific research in general, members of the larger society are obliged to recognize the longer term benefits and risks that may result from the improvement of knowledge and from the development of novel medical, psychotherapeutic, and social procedures.

The principle of beneficence often occupies a well-defined justifying role in many areas of research involving human subjects. An example is found in research involving children. Effective ways of treating childhood diseases and fostering healthy development are benefits that serve to justify research involving children—even when individual research subjects are not direct beneficiaries. Research also makes it possible to avoid the harm that may result from the application of previously accepted routine practices that on closer investigation turn out to be dangerous. But the role of the principle of beneficence is not always so unambiguous. A difficult ethical problem remains, for example, about research that presents more than minimal risk without immediate prospect of direct benefit to the children involved. Some have argued that such research is inadmissible, while others have pointed out that this limit would rule out much research promising great benefit to children in the future. Here again, as with all hard cases, the different claims covered by the principle of beneficence may come into conflict and force difficult choices.

3. Justice—Who ought to receive the benefits of research and bear its burdens? This is a question of justice, in the sense of "fairness in distribution" or "what is deserved." An injustice occurs when some benefit to which a person is entitled is denied without good reason or when some burden is imposed unduly. Another way of conceiving the principle of justice is that equals ought to be treated equally. However, this statement requires explication. Who is equal and who is unequal? What considerations justify departure from equal distribution? Almost all commentators allow that distinctions based on experience, age, deprivation, competence, merit and position do sometimes constitute criteria justifying differential treatment for certain purposes. It is necessary, then, to explain in what respects people should be treated equally. There are several widely accepted formulations of just ways to distribute burdens and benefits. Each formulation mentions some relevant property on the basis of which burdens and benefits should be distributed. These formulations are (1) to each person an equal share, (2) to each person according to individual need, (3) to each person according to individual effort, (4) to each person according to societal contribution, and (5) to each person according to merit.

Questions of justice have long been associated with social practices such as punishment, taxation and political representation. Until recently these questions have not generally been associated with scientific research. However, they are foreshadowed even in the earliest reflections on the ethics of research involving human subjects. For example, during the 19th and early 20th centuries the burdens of serving as research subjects fell largely upon poor ward patients, while the benefits of improved medical care flowed primarily to private patients. Subsequently, the exploitation of unwilling prisoners as research subjects in Nazi concentration camps was condemned as a particularly flagrant injustice. In this country, in the 1940s, the Tuskegee syphilis study used disadvantaged, rural black men to study the untreated course of a disease that is by no means confined to that population. These subjects were deprived of demonstrably effective treatment in order not to interrupt the project, long after such treatment became generally available.

Against this historical background, it can be seen how conceptions of justice are relevant to research involving human subjects. For example, the selection of research subjects needs to be scrutinized in order to determine whether some classes (e.g., welfare patients, particular racial and ethnic minorities, or persons confined to institutions) are being systematically selected simply because of their easy availability, their compromised position, or their manipulability, rather than for reasons directly related to the problem being studied. Finally, whenever research supported by public funds leads to the development of therapeutic devices and procedures, justice demands both that these not provide advantages only to those who can afford them and that such research should not unduly involve persons from groups unlikely to be among the beneficiaries of subsequent applications of the research.

Part C: Applications

Applications of the general principles to the conduct of research leads to consideration of the following requirements: informed consent, risk/benefit assessment, and the selection of subjects of research.

1. Informed Consent—Respect for persons requires that subjects, to the degree that they are capable, be given the opportunity to choose what shall or shall not happen to them. This opportunity is provided when adequate standards for informed consent are satisfied.

While the importance of informed consent is unquestioned, controversy prevails over the nature and possibility of an informed consent. Nonetheless, there is widespread agreement that the consent process can be analyzed as containing three elements: information, comprehension and voluntariness.

Information. Most codes of research establish specific items for disclosure intended to assure that subjects are given sufficient information. These items generally include: the research procedure, their purposes, risks and anticipated benefits, alternative procedures (where therapy is involved), and a statement offering the subject the opportunity to ask questions and to withdraw at any time from the research. Additional items have been proposed, including how subjects are selected, the person responsible for the research, etc.

However, a simple listing of items does not answer the question of what the standard should be for judging how much and what sort of information should be provided. One standard frequently invoked in medical practice, namely the information commonly provided by practitioners in the field or in the locale, is inadequate since research takes place precisely when a common understanding does not exist. Another standard, currently popular in malpractice law, requires the practitioner to reveal the information that reasonable persons would wish to know in order to make a decision regarding their care. This, too, seems insufficient since the research subject, being in essence a volunteer, may wish to know considerably more about risks gratuitously undertaken than do patients who deliver themselves into the hand of a clinician for needed care. It may be that a standard of "the reasonable volunteer" should be proposed: the extent and nature of information should be such that persons, knowing that the procedure is neither necessary for their care nor perhaps fully understood, can decide whether they wish to participate in the furthering of knowledge. Even when some direct benefit to them is anticipated, the subjects should understand clearly the range of risk and the voluntary nature of participation.

A special problem of consent arises where informing subjects of some pertinent aspect of the research is likely to impair the validity of the research. In many cases, it is sufficient to indicate to subjects that they are being invited to participate in research of which some features will not be revealed until the research is concluded. In all cases of research involving incomplete disclosure, such research is justified only if it is clear that (1) incomplete disclosure is truly necessary to accomplish the goals of the research, (2) there are no undisclosed risks to subjects that are more than minimal, and (3) there is an adequate plan for debriefing subjects, when appropriate, and for dissemination of research results to them. Information about risks should never be withheld for the purpose of eliciting the cooperation of subjects, and truthful answers should always be given to direct questions about the research. Care should be taken to distinguish cases in which disclosure would destroy or invalidate the research from cases in which disclosure would simply inconvenience the investigator.

Comprehension. The manner and context in which information is conveyed is as important as the information itself. For example, presenting information in a disorganized and rapid fashion, allowing too little time for consideration or curtailing opportunities for questioning, all may adversely affect a subject's ability to make an informed choice.

Because the subject's ability to understand is a function of intelligence, rationality, maturity and language, it is necessary to adapt the presentation of the information to the subject's capacities. Investigators are responsible for ascertaining that the subject has comprehended the information. While there is always an obligation to ascertain that the information about risk to subjects is complete and adequately comprehended, when the risks are more serious, that obligation increases. On occasion, it may be suitable to give some oral or written tests of comprehension.

Special provision may need to be made when comprehension is severely limited—for example, by conditions of immaturity or mental disability. Each class of subjects that one might consider as incompetent (e.g., infants and young children, mentally disabled patients, the terminally ill and the comatose) should be considered on its own terms. Even for these persons, however, respect requires giving them the opportunity to choose to the extent they are able, whether or not to participate in research. The objections of these subjects to involvement should be honored, unless the research entails providing them a therapy unavailable elsewhere. Respect for persons also requires seeking the permission of other parties in order to protect the subjects from harm. Such persons are thus respected both by acknowledging their own wishes and by the use of third parties to protect them from harm.

The third parties chosen should be those who are most likely to understand the incompetent subject's situation and to act in that person's best interest. The person authorized to act on behalf of the subject should be given an opportunity to observe the research as it proceeds in order to be able to withdraw the subject from the research, if such action appears in the subject's best interest.

Voluntariness. An agreement to participate in research constitutes a valid consent only if voluntarily given. This element of informed consent requires conditions free of coercion and undue influence. Coercion occurs when an overt threat of harm is intentionally presented by one person to another in order to obtain compliance. Undue influence, by contrast, occurs through an offer of an excessive, unwarranted, inappropriate or improper reward or other overture in order to obtain compliance. Also, inducements that would ordinarily be acceptable may become undue influences if the subject is especially vulnerable.

Unjustifiable pressures usually occur when persons in positions of authority or commanding influence—especially where possible sanctions are involved—urge a course of action for a subject. A continuum of such influencing factors exists, however, and it is impossible to state precisely where justifiable persuasion ends and undue influence begins. But undue influence would include actions such as manipulating a person's choice through the controlling influence of a close relative and threatening to withdraw health services to which an individual would otherwise be entitled.

2. Assessment of Risks and Benefits—The assessment of risks and benefits requires a careful arrayal of relevant data, including, in some cases, alternative ways of obtaining the benefits sought in the research. Thus, the assessment presents both an opportunity and a responsibility to gather systematic and comprehensive information about proposed research. For the investigator, it is a means to examine whether the proposed research is properly designed. For a review committee, it is a method for determining whether the risks that will be presented to subjects are justified. For prospective subjects, the assessment will assist the determination whether or not to participate.

The Nature and Scope of Risks and Benefits. The requirement that research be justified on the basis of a favorable risk/benefit assessment bears a close relation to the principle of beneficence, just as the moral requirement that informed consent be obtained is derived primarily from the principle of respect for persons. The term "risk" refers to a possibility that harm may occur. However, when expressions such as "small risk" or "high risk" are used, they usually refer (often ambiguously) both to the chance (probability) of experiencing a harm and the severity (magnitude) of the envisioned harm.

The term "benefit" is used in the research context to refer to something of positive value related to health or welfare. Unlike "risk," "benefit" is not a term that expresses probabilities. Risk is properly contrasted to probability of benefits, and benefits are properly contrasted with harms rather than risks of harm. Accordingly, so-called risk/benefit assessments are concerned with the probabilities and magnitudes of possible harm and anticipated benefits. Many kinds of possible harms and benefits need to be taken into account. There are, for example, risks of psychological harm, physical harm, legal harm, social harm and economic harm and the corresponding benefits. While the most likely types of harms to research subjects are those of psychological or physical pain or injury, other possible kinds should not be overlooked.

Risks and benefits of research may affect the individual subjects, the families of the individual subjects, and society at large (or special groups of subjects in society). Previous codes and Federal regulations have required that risks to subjects be outweighed by the sum of both the anticipated benefit to the subject, if any, and the anticipated benefit to society in the form of knowledge to be gained from the research. In balancing these different elements, the risks and benefits affecting the immediate research subject will normally carry special weight. On the other hand, interests other than those of the subject may on some occasions be sufficient by themselves to justify the risks involved in the research, so long as the subject's rights have been protected. Beneficence thus requires that we protect against risk of harm to subjects and also that we be concerned about the loss of the substantial benefits that might be gained from research.

The Systematic Assessment of Risks and Benefits. It is commonly said that benefits and risks must be "balanced" and shown to be "in a favorable ratio." The metaphorical character of these terms draws attention to the difficulty of making precise judgments. Only on rare occasions will quantitative techniques be available for the scrutiny of research protocols. However, the idea of systematic, nonarbitrary analysis of risks and benefits should be emulated insofar as possible. This ideal requires those making decisions about the justifiability of research to be thorough in the accumulation and assessment of information about all aspects of the research, and to consider alternatives systematically. This procedure renders the assessment of research more rigorous and precise, while making communication between review board members and investigators less subject to misinterpretation, misinformation and conflicting judgments. Thus, there should first be a determination of the validity of the presuppositions of the research; then the nature, probability and magnitude of risk should be distinguished with as much clarity as possible. The method of ascertaining risks should be explicit, especially where there is no alternative to the use of such vague categories as small or slight risk. It should also be determined whether an investigator's estimates of the probability of harm or benefits are reasonable, as judged by known facts or other available studies.

Finally, assessment of the justifiability of research should reflect at least the following considerations: (i) Brutal or inhumane treatment of human subjects is never morally justified. (ii) Risks should be reduced to those necessary to achieve the research objective. It should be determined whether it is in fact necessary to use human subjects at all. Risk can perhaps never be entirely eliminated, but it can often be reduced by careful attention to alternative procedures. (iii) When research involves significant risk of serious impairment, review committees should be extraordinarily insistent on the justification of the risk (looking usually to the likelihood of benefit to the subject—or, in some rare cases, to the manifest voluntariness of the participation). (iv) When vulnerable populations are involved in research, the appropriateness of involving them should itself be demonstrated. A number of variables go into such judgments, including the nature and degree of risk, the condition of the particular population involved, and the nature and level of the anticipated benefits. (v) Relevant risks and benefits must be thoroughly arrayed in documents and procedures used in the informed consent process.

3. Selection of Subjects—Just as the principle of respect for persons finds expression in the requirements for consent, and the principle of beneficence in risk/benefit assessment, the principle of justice gives rise to moral requirements that there be fair procedures and outcomes in the selection of research subjects.

Justice is relevant to the selection of subjects of research at two levels: the social and the individual. Individual justice in the selection of subjects would require that researchers exhibit fairness: thus, they should not offer potentially beneficial research only to some patients who are in their favor or select only "undesirable" persons for risky research. Social justice requires that distinction be drawn between classes of subjects that ought, and ought not, to participate in any particular kind of research, based on the ability of members of that class to bear burdens and on the appropriateness of placing further burdens on already burdened persons. Thus, it can be considered a matter of social justice that there is an order of preference in the selection of classes of subjects (e.g., adults before children) and that some classes of potential subjects (e.g., the institutionalized mentally infirm or prisoners) may be involved as research subjects, if at all, only on certain conditions.

Injustice may appear in the selection of subjects, even if individual subjects are selected fairly by investigators and treated fairly in the course of research. This injustice arises from social, racial, sexual and cultural biases institutionalized in society. Thus, even if individual researchers are treating their research subjects fairly, and even if IRBs [Institutional Review Boards, which approve a research protocol and make sure it is proper] are taking care to assure that subjects are selected fairly within a particular institution, unjust social patterns may nevertheless appear in the overall distribution of the burdens and benefits of research. Although individual institutions or investigators may not be able to resolve a problem that is pervasive in their social setting, they can consider distributive justice in selecting research subjects.

Some populations, especially institutionalized ones, are already burdened in many ways by their infirmities and environments. When research is proposed that involves risks and does not include a therapeutic component, other less burdened classes of persons should be called upon first to accept these risks of research, except where the research is directly related to the specific conditions of the class involved. Also, even though public funds for research may often flow in the same directions as public funds for health care, it seems unfair that populations dependent on public health care constitute a pool of preferred research subjects if more advantaged populations are likely to be the recipients of the benefits.

One special instance of injustice results from the involvement of vulnerable subjects. Certain groups, such as racial minorities, the economically disadvantaged, the very sick, and the institutionalized may continually be sought as research subjects, owing to their ready availability in settings where research is conducted. Given their dependent status and their frequently compromised capacity for free consent, they should be protected against the danger of being involved in research solely for administrative convenience, or because they are easy to manipulate as a result of their illness or socioeconomic condition.

---

1. Since 1945, various codes for the proper and responsible conduct of human experimentation in medical research have been adopted by different organizations. The best known of these codes are the Nuremberg Code of 1947, the Helsinki Declaration of 1964 (revised in 1975), and the 1971 Guidelines (codified into Federal Regulations in 1974) issued by the U.S. Department of Health, Education, and Welfare. Codes for the conduct of social and behavioral research have also been adopted, the best known being that of the American Psychological Association, published in 1973.

2. Although practice usually involves interventions designed solely to enhance the well-being of a particular individual, interventions are sometimes applied to one individual for the enhancement of the well-being of another (e.g., blood donation, skin grafts, organ transplants) or an intervention may have the dual purpose of enhancing the well-being of a particular individual, and, at the same time, providing some benefit to others (e.g., vaccination, which protects both the person who is vaccinated and society generally). The fact that some forms of practice have elements other than immediate benefit to the individual receiving an intervention, however, should not confuse the general distinction between research and practice. Even when a procedure applied in practice may benefit

some other person, it remains an intervention designed to enhance the well-being of a particular individual or groups of individuals; thus, it is practice and need not be reviewed as research.

3. Because the problems related to social experimentation may differ substantially from those of biomedical and behavioral research, the Commission specifically declines to make any policy determination regarding such research at this time. Rather, the Commission believes that the problem ought to be addressed by one of its successor bodies.

THE PRESIDENT DISCUSSES STEM CELL RESEARCH

This is the text of the 2001 address given by President George W. Bush on the topic of federal funding for stem cell research. After several months of deliberation, he announced that he would make funding available for the first time for research involving certain lines of embryo-derived cells. He made the announcement from his ranch in Crawford, Texas.

August 9, 2001

President Discusses Stem Cell Research
The Bush Ranch
Crawford, Texas

8:01 PM CDT

THE PRESIDENT: Good evening. I appreciate you giving me a few minutes of your time tonight so I can discuss with you a complex and difficult issue, an issue that is one of the most profound of our time.

The issue of research involving stem cells derived from human embryos is increasingly the subject of a national debate and dinner table discussions. The issue is confronted every day in laboratories as scientists ponder the ethical ramifications of their work. It is agonized over by parents and many couples as they try to have children, or to save children already born.

The issue is debated within the church, with people of different faiths, even many of the same faith coming to different conclusions. Many people are finding that the more they know about stem cell research, the less certain they are about the right ethical and moral conclusions.

My administration must decide whether to allow federal funds, your tax dollars, to be used for scientific research on stem cells derived from human embryos. A large number of these embryos already exist. They are the product of a process called in vitro fertilization, which helps so many couples conceive children. When doctors match sperm and egg to create life outside the womb, they usually produce more embryos than are planted in the mother. Once a couple successfully has children, or if they are unsuccessful, the additional embryos remain frozen in laboratories.

Some will not survive during long storage; others are destroyed. A number have been donated to science and used to create privately funded stem cell lines. And a few have been implanted in an adoptive mother and born, and are today healthy children.

Based on preliminary work that has been privately funded, scientists believe further research using stem cells offers great promise that could help improve the lives of those who suffer from many terrible diseases—from juvenile diabetes to Alzheimer's, from Parkinson's to spinal cord injuries. And while scientists admit they are not yet certain, they believe stem cells derived from embryos have unique potential.

You should also know that stem cells can be derived from sources other than embryos—from adult cells, from umbilical cords that are discarded after babies are born, from human placenta. And many scientists feel research on these typeof stem cells is also promising. Many patients suffering from a range of diseases are already being helped with treatments developed from adult stem cells.

However, most scientists, at least today, believe that research on embryonic stem cells offer the most promise because these cells have the potential to develop in all of the tissues in the body.

Scientists further believe that rapid progress in this research will come only with federal funds. Federal dollars help attract the best and brightest scientists. They ensure new discoveries are widely shared at the largest number of research facilities and that the research is directed toward the greatest public good.

The United States has a long and proud record of leading the world toward advances in science and medicine that improve human life. And the United States has a long and proud record of upholding the highest standards of ethics as we expand the limits of science and knowledge. Research on embryonic stem cells raises profound ethical questions, because extracting the stem cell destroys the embryo, and thus destroys its potential for life. Like a snowflake, each of these embryos is unique, with the unique genetic potential of an individual human being.

As I thought through this issue, I kept returning to two fundamental questions: First, are these frozen embryos human life, and therefore, something precious to be protected? And second, if they're going to be destroyed anyway, shouldn't they be used for a greater good, for research that has the potential to save and improve other lives?

I've asked those questions and others of scientists, scholars, bioethicists, religious leaders, doctors, researchers, members of Congress, my Cabinet, and my friends. I have read heartfelt letters from many Americans. I have given this issue a great deal of thought, prayer and considerable reflection. And I have found widespread disagreement.

On the first issue, are these embryos human life—well, one researcher told me he believes this five-day-old cluster of cells is not an embryo, not yet an individual, but a pre-embryo. He argued that it has the potential for life, but it is not a life because it cannot develop on its own.

An ethicist dismissed that as a callous attempt at rationalization. Make no mistake, he told me, that cluster of cells is the same way you and I, and all the rest of us, started our lives. One goes with a heavy heart if we use these, he said, because we are dealing with the seeds of the next generation.

And to the other crucial question, if these are going to be destroyed anyway, why not use them for good purpose—I also found different answers. Many argue these embryos are byproducts of a process that helps create life, and we should allow couples to donate them to science so they can be used for good purpose instead of wasting their potential. Others will argue there's no such thing as excess life, and the fact that a living being is going to die does not justify experimenting on it or exploiting it as a natural resource.

At its core, this issue forces us to confront fundamental questions about the beginnings of life and the ends of science. It lies at a difficult moral intersection, juxtaposing the need to protect life in all its phases with the prospect of saving and improving life in all its stages.

As the discoveries of modern science create tremendous hope, they also lay vast ethical mine fields. As the genius of science extends the horizons of what we can do, we increasingly confront complex questions about what we should do. We have arrived at that brave new world that seemed so distant in 1932, when Aldous Huxley wrote about human beings created in test tubes in what he called a "hatchery."

In recent weeks, we learned that scientists have created human embryos in test tubes solely to experiment on them. This is deeply troubling, and a warning sign that should prompt all of us to think through these issues very carefully.

Embryonic stem cell research is at the leading edge of a series of moral hazards. The initial stem cell researcher was at first reluctant to begin his research, fearing it might be used for human cloning. Scientists have already cloned a sheep. Researchers are telling us the next step could be to clone human beings to create individual designer stem cells, essentially to grow another you, to be available in case you need another heart or lung or liver.

I strongly oppose human cloning, as do most Americans. We recoil at the idea of growing human beings for spare body parts, or creating life for our convenience. And while we must devote enormous energy to conquering disease, it is equally important that we pay attention to the moral concerns raised by the new frontier of human embryo stem cell research. Even the most noble ends do not justify any means.

My position on these issues is shaped by deeply held beliefs. I'm a strong supporter of science and technology, and believe they have the potential for incredible good—to improve lives, to save life, to conquer disease. Research offers hope that millions of our loved ones may be cured of a disease and rid of their suffering. I have friends whose children suffer from juvenile diabetes. Nancy Reagan has written me about President Reagan's struggle with Alzheimer's. My own family has confronted the tragedy of childhood leukemia. And, like all Americans, I have great hope for cures.

I also believe human life is a sacred gift from our Creator. I worry about a culture that devalues life, and believe as your President I have an important obligation to foster and encourage respect for life in America and throughout the world. And while we're all hopeful about the potential of this research, no one can be certain that the science will live up to the hope it has generated.

Eight years ago, scientists believed fetal tissue research offered great hope for cures and treatments—yet, the progress to date has not lived up to its initial expectations. Embryonic stem cell research offers both great promise and great peril. So I have decided we must proceed with great care.

As a result of private research, more than 60 genetically diverse stem cell lines already exist. They were created from embryos that have already been destroyed, and they have the ability to regenerate themselves indefinitely, creating ongoing opportunities for research. I have concluded that we should allow federal funds to be used for research on these existing stem cell lines, where the life and death decision has already been made.

Leading scientists tell me research on these 60 lines has great promise that could lead to breakthrough therapies and cures. This allows us to explore the promise and potential of stem cell research without crossing a fundamental moral line, by providing taxpayer funding that would sanction or encourage further destruction of human embryos that have at least the potential for life.

I also believe that great scientific progress can be made through aggressive federal funding of research on umbilical cord, placenta, adult and animal stem cells which do not involve the same moral dilemma. This year, your government will spend $250 million on this important research.

I will also name a President's council to monitor stem cell research, to recommend appropriate guidelines and regulations, and to consider all of the medical and ethical ramifications of biomedical innovation. This council will consist of leading scientists, doctors, ethicists, lawyers, theologians and others, and will be chaired by Dr. Leon Kass, a leading biomedical ethicist from the University of Chicago.

This council will keep us apprised of new developments and give our nation a forum to continue to discuss and evaluate these important issues. As we go forward, I hope we will always be guided by both intellect and heart, by both our capabilities and our conscience.

I have made this decision with great care, and I pray it is the right one.

Thank you for listening. Good night, and God bless America.

END 8:12 P.M. CDT

Source: http://www.whitehouse.gov/news/releases/2001/08/20010809-2.html

NATIONAL INSTITUTES OF HEALTH HUMAN EMBRYONIC STEM CELL REGISTRY

The NIH Human Embryonic Stem Cell Registry lists the derivations of stem cells that are eligible for federal funding. The purpose of the Registry is to provide investigators with a unique NIH Code for each cell line that must be used when applying for NIH funding, as well as contact information to facilitate investigators' acquisition of stem cells. The list of providers and information about their stem cell lines follow. The provider's code gives the name of the line. For example, hES stands for human embryonic stem cell, followed by the identification number of the specific line.

Providers with Lines Available for Shipping
BresaGen, Inc.
Cell Lines Contact Information
Provider's Code: hESBGN-01, hESBGN-02, hESBGN-03, hESBGN-04*
* The cells failed to expand into undifferentiated cell cultures.
BresaGen may have sublines available for shipping. Contact BresaGen for more information about sublines. Subline BG01V is available for shipping

Allan Robins, Ph.D.
Senior Vice President and Chief Scientific Officer
BresaGen, Inc.
111 Riverbend Road
Athens, GA 30605
E-mail: arobins@novocell.com

Cellartis AB
Provider's Code: Sahlgrenska 1, Sahlgrenska 2, Sahlgrenska 3*
* Cell line withdrawn by donor.
Cellartis may have sublines available for shipping. Contact Cellartis for more
information about sublines.
Mikael Englund, Ph.D.
SE-413 46 Göteborg
Sweden
E-mail: mikael.englund@cellartis.com
Web site: http://www.cellartis.com

ES Cell International
Provider's Code: HES-1, HES-2, HES-3, HES-4, HES-5, HES-6
ESCI may have sublines available for shipping. Contact ESCI for more informa-
tion about sublines.
Michael Vovos, IP and Licensing Manager
ES Cell International
41 Science Park Road
04-14/15 The Gemini
Singapore Science Park II
Singapore 117610
E-mail: mvovos@escellinternational.com
Web site: http://www.escellinternational.com
This company also offers hESC training:
http://www.escellinternational.com/research/papers.html
http://www.escellinternational.com/products/trainingsupport.html
http://www.escellinternational.com/products/cellquality.html

MizMedi Hospital—Seoul National University
Provider's Code: Miz-hES1
MizMedi Hospital may have sublines available for shipping. Contact MizMedi
Hospital for more information about sublines.
Sung-il Roh, M.D.
Supervisor
Medical Research Center, MizMedi Hospital
701-4, Naebalsan-dong, Kangseo-ku
Seoul, Korea

E-mail: roh@mizmedi.net
Web site: http://www.mizmedi.com/center/mrclab.asp

Technion–Israel Institute of Technology
Cell Lines Contact Information
Provider's Code: I3, I3.2*, I3.3*, I4, I6, I6.2*, J3*, J3.2*
* These lines are not yet available for shipping.
Technion may have sublines available for shipping. Contact Technion for more information about sublines.
Dr. Joseph Itskovitz, M.D., D.Sc.
Rambam Medical Center
Department of OB/GYN
POB 9602
Haifa 31096
Israel
E-mail: itskovitz@rambam.health.gov.il
Web site: http://www.technion.ac.il

University of California at San Francisco
Department of Obstetrics and Gynecology
Cell Lines Contact Information
Provider's Code: HSF-1, HSF-6

UCSF may have sublines available for shipping. Contact UCSF for more information about sublines.
Box 0720
533 Parnassus Street
San Francisco, CA 94143
E-mail: firpo@itsa.ucsf.edu
Web site: http://escells.ucsf.edu
This provider also offers hESC training:
http://escells.ucsf.edu/Training/Trng.asp

Wisconsin Alumni Research Foundation (WiCell Research Institute)
Cell Lines Contact Information
Provider's Code: H1, H7, H9, H13, H14
WiCell may have sublines available for shipping. Contact WiCell for more information about sublines.
Tammy Torbleau
Secretary, Licensing Department
Wisconsin Alumni Research Foundation (WARF)
P.O. Box 7365
Madison, WI 53707-7365
E-mail: info@wicell.org

Web site: http://www.warf.ws
Web site: http://www.wicell.org
This provider also offers hESC training:
http://www.wicell.org/forresearchers/index.jsp?catid=11
http://www.wicell.org/learn/

For any questions about the NIH Human Embryonic Stem Cell Registry, please
e-mail stemcell@mail.nih.gov or call 301-496-2691.

National Institutes of Health (NIH)
Department of Health and Human Services
9000 Rockville Pike
Bethesda, Maryland 20892

Roe v. Wade

This case appeared before the U.S. Supreme Court as a challenge to an 1859
Texas abortion law that declared abortion illegal except to save the life of the
mother. The Court's decision of 22 January 1973 invalidated all state laws
restricting abortion in the first trimester. Argument of the majority was presented
by Justice Harry Blackmun. The dissenting opinion was written by Justice
William Rehnquist.

410 U.S. 113

SUPREME COURT OF THE UNITED STATES

ROE, ET AL.

v.

WADE,

DISTRICT ATTORNEY OF DALLAS COUNTY

January 22, 1973

APPEAL FROM THE UNITED STATES DISTRICT COURT
FOR THE NORTHERN DISTRICT OF TEXAS

No. 70-18.

———

Argued December 13, 1971
Reargued October 11, 1972
Decided January 22, 1973

BLACKMUN, J., delivered the opinion of the Court, in which BURGER, C. J., and DOUGLAS, BRENNAN, STEWART, MARSHALL, and POWELL, JJ., joined. BURGER, C. J., *post,* p. 207, DOUGLAS, J., *post,* p. 209, and STEWART, J., *post,* p. 167, filed concurring opinions. WHITE, J., filed a dissenting opinion, in which REHNQUIST, J., joined, *post,* p. 221. REHNQUIST, J., filed a dissenting opinion, *post,* p. 171.

A pregnant single woman (Roe) brought a class action challenging the constitutionality of the Texas criminal abortion laws, which proscribe procuring or attempting an abortion except on medical advice for the purpose of saving the mother's life. A licensed physician (Hallford), who had two state abortion prosecutions pending against him, was permitted to intervene. A childless married couple (the Does), the wife not being pregnant, separately attacked the laws, basing alleged injury on the future possibilities of contraceptive failure, pregnancy, unpreparedness for parenthood, and impairment of the wife's health. A three-judge District Court, which consolidated the actions, held that Roe and Hallford, and members of their classes, had standing to sue and presented justiciable controversies. Ruling that declaratory, though not injunctive, relief was warranted, the court declared the abortion statutes void as vague and overbroadly infringing those plaintiffs' Ninth and Fourteenth Amendment rights. The court ruled the Does' complaint not justiciable. Appellants directly appealed to this Court on the injunctive rulings, and appellee cross-appealed from the District Court's grant of declaratory relief to Roe and Hallford.

- *Held:*
- 1. While 28 U.S.C. §1253 authorizes no direct appeal to this Court from the grant or denial of declaratory relief alone, review is not foreclosed when the case is properly before the Court on appeal from specific denial of injunctive relief and the arguments as to both injunctive and declaratory relief are necessarily identical.
- 2. Roe has standing to sue; the Does and Hallford do not.
  - (a) Contrary to appellee's contention, the natural termination of Roe's pregnancy did not moot her suit. Litigation involving pregnancy, which is "capable of repetition, yet evading review," is an exception to the usual federal rule that an actual controversy [p114] must exist at review stages and not simply when the action is initiated. [ ]
  - (b) The District Court correctly refused injunctive, but erred in granting declaratory, relief to Hallford, who alleged no federally protected right not assertable as a defense against the good-faith

state prosecutions pending against him. *Samuels* v. *Mackell*, 401 U.S. 66.

o (c) The Does' complaint, based as it is on contingencies, any one or more of which may not occur, is too speculative to present an actual case or controversy.

• 3. State criminal abortion laws, like those involved here, that except from criminality only a life-saving procedure on the mother's behalf without regard to the stage of her pregnancy and other interests involved violate the Due Process Clause of the Fourteenth Amendment, which protects against state action the right to privacy, including a woman's qualified right to terminate her pregnancy. Though the State cannot override that right, it has legitimate interests in protecting both the pregnant woman's health and the potentiality of human life, each of which interests grows and reaches a "compelling" point at various stages of the woman's approach to term.

o (a) For the stage prior to approximately the end of the first trimester, the abortion decision and its effectuation must be left to the medical judgment of the pregnant woman's attending physician.

o (b) For the stage subsequent to approximately the end of the first trimester, the State, in promoting its interest in the health of the mother, may, if it chooses, regulate the abortion procedure in ways that are reasonably related to maternal health.

o (c) For the stage subsequent to viability the State, in promoting its interest in the potentiality of human life, may, if it chooses, regulate, and even proscribe, abortion except where necessary, in appropriate medical judgment, for the preservation of the life or health of the mother.

• 4. The State may define the term "physician" to mean only a physician currently licensed by the State, and may proscribe any abortion by a person who is not a physician as so defined.

• 5. It is unnecessary to decide the injunctive relief issue since the Texas authorities will doubtless fully recognize the Court's ruling [p115] that the Texas criminal abortion statutes are unconstitutional.

314 F. Supp. 1217, affirmed in part and reversed in part.

Sarah Weddington reargued the cause for appellants. With her on the briefs were *Roy Lucas, Fred Bruner, Roy L. Merrill, Jr.,* and *Norman Dorsen.*

Robert C. Flowers, Assistant Attorney General of Texas, argued the cause for appellee on the reargument. *Jay Floyd,* Assistant Attorney General, argued the cause for appellee on the original argument. With them on the brief were *Crawford C. Martin,* Attorney General, *Nola White,* First Assistant Attorney General, *Alfred Walker,* Executive Assistant Attorney General, *Henry Wade,* and *John B. Tolle.**

[Blackmun, J.—Opinion of the Court]
[Stewart, J.—Concurring opinion]
[Rehnquist, J.—Dissenting opinion]
[Burger, C. J.—Concurring (both *Roe* and *Doe*)]
[Douglas, J.—Concurring (both *Roe* and *Doe*)]
[White, J.—Dissenting (both *Roe* and *Doe*)]

[Transcript of Oral Arguments (#1) (#2)]

Blackmun, J.—Opinion of the Court

[p116] MR. JUSTICE BLACKMUN delivered the opinion of the Court.

This Texas federal appeal and its Georgia companion, *Doe v. Bolton, post,* p. 179, present constitutional challenges to state criminal abortion legislation. The Texas statutes under attack here are typical of those that have been in effect in many States for approximately a century. The Georgia statutes, in contrast, have a modern cast and are a legislative product that, to an extent at least, obviously reflects the influences of recent attitudinal change, of advancing medical knowledge and techniques, and of new thinking about an old issue.

We forthwith acknowledge our awareness of the sensitive and emotional nature of the abortion controversy, of the vigorous opposing views, even among physicians, and of the deep and seemingly absolute convictions that the subject inspires. One's philosophy, one's experiences, one's exposure to the raw edges of human existence, one's religious training, one's attitudes toward life and family and their values, and the moral standards one establishes and seeks to observe, are all likely to influence and to color one's thinking and conclusions about abortion.

In addition, population growth, pollution, poverty, and racial overtones tend to complicate and not to simplify the problem.

Our task, of course, is to resolve the issue by constitutional measurement, free of emotion and of predilection. We seek earnestly to do this, and, because we do, we [p117] have inquired into, and in this opinion place some emphasis upon, medical and medical-legal history and what that history reveals about man's attitudes toward the abortion procedure over the centuries. We bear in mind, too, Mr. Justice Holmes' admonition in his now-vindicated dissent in *Lochner* v. *New York,* 198 U.S. 45, 76 (1905):

> • "[The Constitution] is made for people of fundamentally differing views, and the accident of our finding certain opinions natural and

familiar or novel and even shocking ought not to conclude our judgment upon the question whether statutes embodying them conflict with the Constitution of the United States."

I

The Texas statutes that concern us here are Arts. 1191–1194 and 1196 of the State's Penal Code.[1] These make it a crime to "procure an abortion," as therein [p118] defined, or to attempt one, except with respect to "an abortion procured or attempted by medical advice for the purpose of saving the life of the mother." Similar statutes are in existence in a majority of the States.[2]

[p119] Texas first enacted a criminal abortion statute in 1854. Texas Laws 1854 c. 49, §1, set forth in 3 H. Gammel, Laws of Texas 1502 (1898). This was soon modified into language that has remained substantially unchanged to the present time. See Texas Penal Code of 1857, c. 7 Arts. 531–536; G. Paschal, Laws of Texas, Arts. 2192–2197 (1866); Texas Rev. Stat., c. 8, Arts. 536–541 (1879); Texas Rev. Crim. Stat., Arts. 1071–1076 (1911). The final article in each of these compilations provided the same exception, as does the present Article 1196, for an abortion by "medical advice for the purpose of saving the life of the mother."[3][p120]

II

Jane Roe,[4] a single woman who was residing in Dallas County, Texas, instituted this federal action in March 1970 against the District Attorney of the county. She sought a declaratory judgment that the Texas criminal abortion statutes were unconstitutional on their face, and an injunction restraining the defendant from enforcing the statutes.

Roe alleged that she was unmarried and pregnant; that she wished to terminate her pregnancy by an abortion "performed by a competent, licensed physician, under safe clinical conditions"; that she was unable to get a "legal" abortion in Texas because her life did not appear to be threatened by the continuation of her pregnancy; and that she could not afford to travel to another jurisdiction in order to secure a legal abortion under safe conditions. She claimed that the Texas statutes were unconstitutionally vague and that they abridged her right of personal privacy, protected by the First, Fourth, Fifth, Ninth, and Fourteenth Amendments. By an amendment to her complaint Roe purported to sue "on behalf of herself and all other women" similarly situated.

James Hubert Hallford, a licensed physician, sought and was granted leave to intervene in Roe's action. In his complaint he alleged that he had been arrested previously for violations of the Texas abortion statutes and [p121] that two such prosecutions were pending against him. He described conditions of patients who came to him seeking abortions, and he claimed that for many cases he, as a physician, was unable to determine whether they fell within or outside the exception recognized by Article 1196. He alleged that, as a consequence, the statutes were vague and uncertain, in violation of the Fourteenth Amendment, and that they violated his own and his patients' rights to privacy in the doctor–patient relationship and his own right to practice medicine, rights he claimed were guaranteed by the First, Fourth, Fifth, Ninth, and Fourteenth Amendments.

John and Mary Doe,[5] a married couple, filed a companion complaint to that of Roe. They also named the District Attorney as defendant, claimed like constitutional deprivations, and sought declaratory and injunctive relief. The Does alleged that they were a childless couple; that Mrs. Doe was suffering from a "neuralchemical" disorder; that her physician had "advised her to avoid pregnancy until such time as her condition has materially improved" (although a pregnancy at the present time would not present "a serious risk" to her life); that, pursuant to medical advice, she had discontinued use of birth control pills; and that if she should become pregnant, she would want to terminate the pregnancy by an abortion performed by a competent, licensed physician under safe, clinical conditions. By an amendment to their complaint, the Does purported to sue "on behalf of themselves and all couples similarly situated."

The two actions were consolidated and heard together by a duly convened three-judge district court. The suits thus presented the situations of the pregnant single woman, the childless couple, with the wife not pregnant, [p122] and the licensed practicing physician, all joining in the attack on the Texas criminal abortion statutes. Upon the filing of affidavits, motions were made for dismissal and for summary judgment. The court held that Roe and members of her class, and Dr. Hallford, had standing to sue and presented justiciable controversies, but that the Does had failed to allege facts sufficient to state a present controversy and did not have standing. It concluded that, with respect to the requests for a declaratory judgment, abstention was not warranted. On the merits, the District Court held that the "fundamental right of single women and married persons to choose whether to have children is protected by the Ninth Amendment, through the Fourteenth Amendment," and that the Texas criminal abortion statutes were void on their face because they were both unconstitutionally vague and constituted an overbroad infringement of the plaintiffs" Ninth Amendment rights. The court then held that abstention was warranted with respect to the requests for an injunction. It therefore dismissed the Does' complaint, declared the abortion statutes void, and dismissed the application for injunctive relief. 314 F. Supp. 1217, 1225 (ND Tex. 1970).

The plaintiffs Roe and Doe and the intervenor Hallford, pursuant to 28 U.S.C. §1253, have appealed to this Court from that part of the District Court's judgment denying the injunction. The defendant District Attorney has purported tocross-appeal, pursuant to the same statute, from the court's grant of declaratory relief to Roe and Hallford. Both sides also have taken protective appeals to the United States Court of Appeals for the Fifth Circuit. That court ordered the appeals held in abeyance pending decision here. We postponed decision on jurisdiction to the hearing on the merits. 402 U.S. 941 (1971). [p123]

III

It might have been preferable if the defendant, pursuant to our Rule 20, had presented to us a petition for certiorari before judgment in the Court of Appeals with respect to the granting of the plaintiffs' prayer for declaratory relief. Our decisions in *Mitchell* v. *Donovan,* 398 U.S. 427 (1970), and *Gunn* v. *University Committee,* 399 U.S. 383 (1970), are to the effect that §1253 does not authorize an appeal to this Court from the grant or denial of declaratory relief alone. We conclude, nevertheless, that those decisions do not foreclose our review of both the injunctive and the declaratory aspects of a case of this kind when it is properly here, as this one is, on appeal under §1253 from specific denial of injunctive relief, and the arguments as to both aspects are necessarily identical. See *Carter* v. *Jury Comm'n,* 396 U.S. 320 (1970); *Florida Lime Growers* v. *Jacobsen,* 362 U.S. 73, 80–81 (1960). It would be destructive of time and energy for all concerned were we to rule otherwise. Cf. *Doe* v. *Bolton, post,* p. 179.

IV

We are next confronted with issues of justiciability, standing, and abstention. Have Roe and the Does established that "personal stake in the outcome of the controversy," *Baker* v. *Carr,* 369 U.S. 186, 204 (1962), that insures that "the dispute sought to be adjudicated will be presented in an adversary context and in a form historically viewed as capable of judicial resolution," *Flast* v. *Cohen,* 392 U.S. 83, 101 (1968), and *Sierra Club* v. *Morton,* 405 U.S. 727, 732 (1972)? And what effect did the pendency of criminal abortion charges against Dr. Hallford in state court have upon the propriety of the federal court's granting relief to him as a plaintiff-intervenor? [p124]

A. *Jane Roe.* Despite the use of the pseudonym, no suggestion is made that Roe is a fictitious person. For purposes of her case, we accept as true, and as established, her existence; her pregnant state, as of the inception of her suit in March 1970 and as late as May 21 of that year when she filed an alias affidavit with the District Court; and her inability to obtain a legal abortion in Texas.

Viewing Roe's case as of the time of its filing and thereafter until as late as May, there can be little dispute that it then presented a case or controversy and that, wholly apart from the class aspects, she, as a pregnant single woman thwarted by the Texas criminal abortion laws, had standing to challenge those statutes. *Abele* v. *Markle,* 452 F.2d 1121, 1125 (CA2 1971); *Crossen* v. *Breckenridge,* 446 F.2d

833, 838–839 (CA6 1971); *Poe* v. *Menghini,* 339 F. Supp. 986, 990–991 (Kan. 1972). See *Truax* v. *Raich,* 239 U.S. 33 (1915). Indeed, we do not read the appellee's brief as really asserting anything to the contrary. The "logical nexus between the status asserted and the claim sought to be adjudicated," *Flast* v. *Cohen,* 392 U.S., at 102, and the necessary degree of contentiousness, *Golden* v. *Zwickler,* 394 U.S. 103 (1969), are both present.

The appellee notes, however, that the record does not disclose that Roe was pregnant at the time of the District Court hearing on May 22, 1970,[6] or on the following June 17 when the court's opinion and judgment were filed. And he suggests that Roe's case must now be moot because she and all other members of her class are no longer subject to any 1970 pregnancy. [p125]

The usual rule in federal cases is that an actual controversy must exist at stages of appellate or certiorari review, and not simply at the date the action is initiated. *United States* v. *Munsingwear, Inc.,* 340 U.S. 36 (1950); *Golden* v. *Zwickler, supra; SEC* v. *Medical Committee for Human Rights,* 404 U.S. 403 (1972).

But when, as here, pregnancy is a significant fact in the litigation, the normal 266-day human gestation period is so short that the pregnancy will come to term before the usual appellate process is complete. If that termination makes a case moot, pregnancy litigation seldom will survive much beyond the trial stage, and appellate review will be effectively denied. Our law should not be that rigid. Pregnancy often comes more than once to the same woman, and in the general population, if man is to survive, it will always be with us. Pregnancy provides a classic justification for a conclusion of nonmootness. It truly could be "capable of repetition, yet evading review." *Southern Pacific Terminal Co.* v. *ICC,* 219 U.S. 498, 515 (1911). See *Moore* v. *Ogilvie,* 394 U.S. 814, 816 (1969); *Carroll* v. *Princess Anne,* 393 U.S. 175, 178–179 (1968); *United States* v. *W. T. Grant Co.,* 345 U.S. 629, 632–633 (1953).

We, therefore, agree with the District Court that Jane Roe had standing to undertake this litigation, that she presented a justiciable controversy, and that the termination of her 1970 pregnancy has not rendered her case moot.

B. *Dr. Hallford.* The doctor's position is different. He entered Roe's litigation as a plaintiff-intervenor, alleging in his complaint that he:

"[I]n the past has been arrested for violating the Texas Abortion Laws and at the present time stands charged by indictment with violating said laws in the Criminal District Court of Dallas County, Texas to-wit: (1) The State of Texas vs. James H. Hallford, No. C-69-5307-IH, and (2) The State of Texas vs. [p126] James H. Hallford, No. C-69-2524-H. In both cases the defendant is charged with abortion...."

In his application for leave to intervene, the doctor made like representations as to the abortion charges pending in the state court. These representations were also repeated in the affidavit he executed and filed in support of his motion for summary judgment.

Dr. Hallford is, therefore, in the position of seeking, in a federal court, declaratory and injunctive relief with respect to the same statutes under which he stands charged in criminal prosecutions simultaneously pending in state court. Although he stated that he has been arrested in the past for violating the State's abortion laws, he makes no allegation of any substantial and immediate threat to any federally protected right that cannot be asserted in his defense against the state prosecutions. Neither is there any allegation of harassment or bad-faith prosecution. In order to escape the rule articulated in the cases cited in the next paragraph of this opinion that, absent harassment and bad faith, a defendant in a pending state criminal case cannot affirmatively challenge in federal court the statutes under which the State is prosecuting him, Dr. Hallford seeks to distinguish his status as a present state defendant from his status as a "potential future defendant" and to assert only the latter for standing purposes here.

We see no merit in that distinction. Our decision in *Samuels v. Mackell,* 401 U.S. 66 (1971), compels the conclusion that the District Court erred when it granted declaratory relief to Dr. Hallford instead of refraining from so doing. The court, of course, was correct in refusing to grant injunctive relief to the doctor. The reasons supportive of that action, however, are those expressed in *Samuels* v. *Mackell, supra,* and in *Younger v.* [p127] *Harris,* 401 U.S. 37 (1971); *Boyle v. Landry,* 401 U.S. 77 (1971); *Perez* v. *Ledesma,* 401 U.S. 82 (1971); and *Byrne* v. *Karalexis,* 401 U.S. 216 (1971). See also *Dombrowski* v. *Pfister,* 380 U.S. 479 (1965). We note, in passing, that *Younger* and its companion cases were decided after the three-judge District Court decision in this case.

Dr. Hallford's complaint in intervention, therefore, is to be dismissed.[7] He is remitted to his defenses in the state criminal proceedings against him. We reverse the judgment of the District Court insofar as it granted Dr. Hallford relief and failed to dismiss his complaint in intervention.

C. *The Does.* In view of our ruling as to Roe's standing in her case, the issue of the Does' standing in their case has little significance. The claims they assert are essentially the same as those of Roe, and they attack the same statutes. Nevertheless, we briefly note the Does' posture.

Their [p128] pleadings present them as a childless married couple, the woman not being pregnant, who have no desire to have children at this time because of their having received medical advice that Mrs. Doe should avoid pregnancy, and for "other highly personal reasons." But they "fear. . . they may face the prospect of becoming parents." And if pregnancy ensues, they "would want to terminate" it by an abortion. They assert an inability to obtain an abortion legally in Texas and, consequently, the prospect of obtaining an illegal abortion there or of going outside Texas to some place where the procedure could be obtained legally and competently.

We thus have as plaintiffs a married couple who have, as their asserted immediate and present injury, only an alleged "detrimental effect upon [their] marital happiness" because they are forced to "the choice of refraining from normal sexual relations or of endangering Mary Doe's health through a possible pregnancy." Their claim is that sometime in the future Mrs. Doe might become pregnant because of possible failure of contraceptive measures, and at that time in the future she might want an abortion that might then be illegal under the Texas statutes.

This very phrasing of the Does' position reveals its speculative character. Their alleged injury rests on possible future contraceptive failure, possible future pregnancy, possible future unpreparedness for parenthood, and possible future impairment of health. Any one or more of these several possibilities may not take place and all may not combine. In the Does' estimation, these possibilities might have some real or imagined impact upon their marital happiness. But we are not prepared to say that the bare allegation of so indirect an injury is sufficient to present an actual case or controversy. *Younger* v. *Harris,* 401 U.S., at 41–42; *Golden* v. *Zwickler,* 394 U.S., at 109–110; *Abele* v. *Markle,* 452 F. 2d, at 1124–1125; *Crossen* v. *Breckenridge,* 446 F. 2d, at 839. The Does' claim falls far short of those resolved otherwise in the cases that the Does urge upon us, namely, *Investment Co. Institute* v. *Camp,* 401 U.S. 617 (1971); *Data Processing Service* v. *Camp,* 397 U.S. 150 (1970); [p129] and *Epperson* v. *Arkansas,* 393 U.S. 97 (1968). See also *Truax v. Raich,* 239 U.S. 33 (1915).

The Does therefore are not appropriate plaintiffs in this litigation. Their complaint was properly dismissed by the District Court, and we affirm that dismissal.

---

1. "Article 1191. Abortion

"If any person shall designedly administer to a pregnant woman or knowingly procure to be administered with her consent any drug or medicine, or shall use towards her any violence or means whatever externally or internally applied, and thereby procure an abortion, he shall be confined in the penitentiary not less than two nor more than five years; if it be done without her consent, the punishment shall be doubled. By 'abortion' is meant that the life of the fetus or embryo shall be destroyed in the woman's womb or that a premature birth thereof be caused.

"Art. 1192. Furnishing the means

"Whoever furnishes the means for procuring an abortion knowing the purpose intended is guilty as an accomplice.

"Art. 1193. Attempt at abortion

"If the means used shall fail to produce an abortion, the offender is nevertheless guilty of an attempt to produce abortion, provided it be shown that such means were calculated to produce that result, and shall be fined not less than one hundred nor more than one thousand dollars.

"Art. 1194. Murder in producing abortion

"If the death of the mother is occasioned by an abortion so produced or by an attempt to effect the same it is murder."

"Art. 1196. By medical advice

"Nothing in this chapter applies to an abortion procured or attempted by medical advice for the purpose of saving the life of the mother."

The foregoing Articles, together with Art. 1195, compose Chapter 9 of Title 15 of the Penal Code. Article 1195, not attacked here, reads:

"Art. 1195. Destroying unborn child

"Whoever shall during parturition of the mother destroy the vitality or life in a child in a state of being born and before actual birth, which child would otherwise have been born alive, shall be confined in the penitentiary for life or for not less than five years."

2. Ariz. Rev. Stat. Ann. §13-211 (1956); Conn. Pub. Act No. 1 (May 1972 special session) (in 4 Conn. Leg. Serv. 677 (1972)), and Conn. Gen. Stat. Rev. §§53-29, 53-30 (1968) (or unborn child); Idaho Code §18-601 (1948); Ill. Rev. Stat., c. 38, §23-1 (1971); Ind. Code §35-1-58-1 (1971); Iowa Code §701.1 (1971); Ky. Rev. Stat. §436.020 (1962); La. Rev. Stat. §37:1285(6) (1964) (loss of medical license) (but see §14:87 (Supp. 1972) containing no exception for the life of the mother under the criminal statute); Me. Rev. Stat. Ann., Tit. 17, §51 (1964); Mass. Gen. Laws Ann., c. 272, §19 (1970) (using the term "unlawfully," construed to exclude an abortion to save the mother's life, *Kudish* v. *Bd. of Registration,* 356 Mass. 98, 248 N.E.2d 264 (1969)); Mich. Comp. Laws §750.14 (1948); Minn. Stat. §617.18 (1971); Mo. Rev. Stat. §559.100 (1969); Mont. Rev. Codes Ann. §94-401 (1969); Neb. Rev. Stat. §28-405 (1964); Nev. Rev. Stat. §200.220 (1967); N.H. Rev. Stat. Ann. §585:13 (1955); N.J. Stat. Ann. §2A:87-1 (1969) ("without lawful justification"); N.D. Cent. Code §§12-25-01, 12-25-02 (1960); Ohio Rev. Code Ann. §2901.16 (1953); Okla. Stat. Ann., Tit. 21, §861 (1972–1973 Supp.); Pa. Stat.

Ann., Tit. 18, §§4718, 4719 (1963) ("unlawful"); R.I. Gen. Laws Ann. §11-3-1 (1969); S.D. Comp. Laws Ann. §22-17-1 (1967); Tenn. Code Ann. §§39-301, 39–302 (1956); Utah Code Ann. §§76-2-1, 76-2-2 (1953); Vt. Stat. Ann., Tit. 13, §101 (1958); W. Va. Code Ann. §61-2-8 (1966); Wis. Stat. §940.04 (1969); Wyo. Stat. Ann. §§6-77, 6-78 (1957).

3. Long ago, a suggestion was made that the Texas statutes were unconstitutionally vague because of definitional deficiencies. The Texas Court of Criminal Appeals disposed of that suggestion peremptorily, saying only,

"It is also insisted in the motion in arrest of judgment that the statute is unconstitutional and void in that it does not sufficiently define or describe the offense of abortion. We do not concur in respect to this question." *Jackson* v. *State,* 55 Tex. Cr. R. 79, 89, 115 S.W. 262, 268 (1908).

The same court recently has held again that the State's abortion statutes are not unconstitutionally vague or overbroad. *Thompson* v. *State* (Ct. Crim. App. Tex. 1971), appeal docketed, No. 71-1200. The court held that "the State of Texas has a compelling interest to protect fetal life"; that Art. 1191 "is designed to protect fetal life"; that the Texas homicide statutes, particularly Art. 1205 of the Penal Code, are intended to protect a person "in existence by actual birth" and thereby implicitly recognize other human life that is not "in existence by actual birth"; that the definition of human life is for the legislature and not the courts; that Art. 1196 "is more definite than the District of Columbia statute upheld in [*United States* v.] *Vuitch*" (402 U.S. 62); and that the Texas statute "is not vague and indefinite or overbroad." A physician's abortion conviction was affirmed.

In *Thompson,* n. 2, the court observed that any issue as to the burden of proof under the exemption of Art. 1196 "is not before us." But see *Veevers* v. *State,* 172 Tex. Cr. R. 162, 168–169, 354 S.W.2d 161, 166–167 (1962). Cf. *United States* v. *Vuitch,* 402 U.S. 62, 69–71 (1971).

4. The name is a pseudonym.

5. These names are pseudonyms.

6. The appellee twice states in his brief that the hearing before the District Court was held on July 22, 1970. Brief for Appellee 13. The docket entries, App. 2, and the transcript, App. 76, reveal this to be an error. The July date appears to be the time of the reporter's transcription.

7. We need not consider what different result, if any, would follow if Dr. Hallford's intervention were on behalf of a class. His complaint in intervention does not purport to assert a class suit and makes no reference to any class apart from an allegation that he "and others similarly situated" must necessarily guess at the meaning of Art. 1196. His application for leave to intervene goes somewhat further, for it

asserts that plaintiff Roe does not adequately protect the interest of the doctor "and the class of people who are physicians...[and] the class of people who are...patients...."

The leave application, however, is not the complaint. Despite the District Court's statement to the contrary, 314 F. Supp., at 1225, we fail to perceive the essentials of a class suit in the Hallford complaint.

Rehnquist, J.—Dissenting

MR. JUSTICE REHNQUIST, dissenting.

The Court's opinion brings to the decision of this troubling question both extensive historical fact and a wealth of legal scholarship. While the opinion thus commands my respect, I find myself nonetheless in fundamental disagreement with those parts of it that invalidate the Texas statute in question, and therefore dissent.

I

The Court's opinion decides that a State may impose virtually no restriction on the performance of abortions during the first trimester of pregnancy. Our previous decisions indicate that a necessary predicate for such an opinion is a plaintiff who was in her first trimester of pregnancy at some time during the pendency of her lawsuit. While a party may vindicate his own constitutional rights, he may not seek vindication for the rights of others. *Moose Lodge* v. *Irvis,* 407 U.S. 163 (1972); *Sierra Club* v. *Morton*, 405 U.S. 727 (1972). The Court's statement of facts in this case makes clear, however, that the record in no way indicates the presence of such a plaintiff. We know only that plaintiff Roe at the time of filing her complaint was a pregnant woman; for aught that appears in this record, she may have been in her last trimester of pregnancy as of the date the complaint was filed.

Nothing in the Court's opinion indicates that Texas might not constitutionally apply its proscription of abortion as written to a woman in that stage of pregnancy. Nonetheless, the Court uses her complaint against the Texas statute as a fulcrum for deciding that States may [p172] impose virtually no restrictions on medical abortions performed during the *first* trimester of pregnancy. In deciding such a hypothetical lawsuit, the Court departs from the longstanding admonition that it should never "formulate a rule of constitutional law broader than is required by the precise facts to which it is to be applied." *Liverpool, New York & Philalelphia S. S. Co.* v. *Commissioners of Emigration*, 113 U.S. 33, 39 (1885). See also *Ashwander* v. *TVA*, 297 U.S. 288, 345 (1936) (Brandeis, J., concurring).

II

Even if there were a plaintiff in this case capable of litigating the issue which the Court decides, I would reach a conclusion opposite to that reached by the Court. I have difficulty in concluding, as the Court does, that the right of "privacy" is involved in this case. Texas, by the statute here challenged, bars the performance of a medical abortion by a licensed physician on a plaintiff such as Roe. A transaction resulting in an operation such as this is not "private" in the ordinary usage of that word. Nor is the "privacy" that the Court finds here even a distant relative of the freedom from searches and seizures protected by the Fourth Amendment to the Constitution, which the Court has referred to as embodying a right to privacy. *Katz* v. *United States,* 389 U.S. 347 (1967).

If the Court means by the term "privacy" no more than that the claim of a person to be free from unwanted state regulation of consensual transactions may be a form of "liberty" protected by the Fourteenth Amendment, there is no doubt that similar claims have been upheld in our earlier decisions on the basis of that liberty. I agree with the statement of MR. JUSTICE STEWART in his concurring opinion that the "liberty," against deprivation of which without due process the Fourteenth [p173] Amendment protects, embraces more than the rights found in the Bill of Rights. But that liberty is not guaranteed absolutely against deprivation, only against deprivation without due process of law. The test traditionally applied in the area of social and economic legislation is whether or not a law such as that challenged has a rational relation to a valid state objective. *Williamson* v. *Lee Optical Co.,* 348 U.S. 483, 491 (1955). The Due Process Clause of the Fourteenth Amendment undoubtedly does place a limit, albeit a broad one, on legislative power to enact laws such as this. If the Texas statute were to prohibit an abortion even where the mother's life is in jeopardy, I have little doubt that such a statute would lack a rational relation to a valid state objective under the test stated in *Williamson, supra.* But the Court's sweeping invalidation of any restrictions on abortion during the first trimester is impossible to justify under that standard, and the conscious weighing of competing factors that the Court's opinion apparently substitutes for the established test is far more appropriate to a legislative judgment than to a judicial one.

The Court eschews the history of the Fourteenth Amendment in its reliance on the "compelling state interest" test. See *Weber* v. *Aetna Casualty & Surety Co.,* 406 U.S. 164, 179 (1972) (dissenting opinion). But the Court adds a new wrinkle to this test by transposing it from the legal considerations associated with the Equal Protection Clause of the Fourteenth Amendment to this case arising under the Due Process Clause of the Fourteenth Amendment. Unless I misapprehend the consequences of this transplanting of the "compelling state interest test," the Court's opinion will accomplish the seemingly impossible feat of leaving this area of the law more confused than it found it. [p174]

While the Court's opinion quotes from the dissent of Mr. Justice Holmes in *Lochner* v. *New York,* 198 U.S. 45, 74 (1905), the result it reaches is more closely attuned to the majority opinion of Mr. Justice Peckham in that case. As in *Lochner* and similar cases applying substantive due process standards to economic and social welfare legislation, the adoption of the compelling state interest standard will inevitably require this Court to examine the legislative policies and pass on the wisdom of these policies in the very process of deciding whether a particular state interest put forward may or may not be "compelling." The decision here to break pregnancy into three distinct terms and to outline the permissible restrictions the State may impose in each one, for example, partakes more of judicial legislation than it does of a determination of the intent of the drafters of the Fourteenth Amendment.

The fact that a majority of the States reflecting, after all, the majority sentiment in those States, have had restrictions on abortions for at least a century is a strong indication, it seems to me, that the asserted right to an abortion is not "so rooted in the traditions and conscience of our people as to be ranked as fundamental," *Snyder* v. *Massachusetts,* 291 U.S. 97, 105 (1934). Even today, when society's views on abortion are changing, the very existence of the debate is evidence that the "right" to an abortion is not so universally accepted as the appellant would have us believe.

To reach its result the Court necessarily has had to find within the scope of the Fourteenth Amendment a right that was apparently completely unknown to the drafters of the Amendment. As early as 1821, the first state law dealing directly with abortion was enacted by the Connecticut Legislature. Conn. Stat., Tit. 22, §§14, 16. By the time of the adoption of the Fourteenth [p175] Amendment in 1868, there were at least 36 laws enacted by state or territorial legislatures limiting abortion.[1] While many States have amended or updated [p176] their laws, 21 of the laws on the books in 1868 remain in effect today.[2] Indeed, the Texas statute struck down today was, as the majority notes, first enacted in 1857 [p177] and "has remained substantially unchanged to the present time." *Ante,* at 119.

There apparently was no question concerning the validity of this provision or of any of the other state statutes when the Fourteenth Amendment was adopted. The only conclusion possible from this history is that the drafters did not intend to have the Fourteenth Amendment withdraw from the States the power to legislate with respect to this matter.

III

Even if one were to agree that the case that the Court decides were here, and that the enunciation of the substantive constitutional law in the Court's opinion were proper, the actual disposition of the case by the Court is still difficult to justify. The Texas statute is struck down in *toto,* even though the Court apparently concedes that at later periods of pregnancy Texas might impose these selfsame statutory limitations on abortion. My understanding of past practice is that a statute found [p178] to be invalid as applied to a particular plaintiff, but not unconstitutional as a whole, is not simply "struck down" but is, instead, declared unconstitutional as applied to the fact situation before the Court. *Yick Wo* v. *Hopkins,* 118 U.S.356 (1886); *Street* v. *New York,* 394 U.S.576 (1969).

For all of the foregoing reasons, I respectfully dissent.

---

1. Jurisdictions having enacted abortion laws prior to the adoption of the Fourteenth Amendment in 1868:

1. Alabama—Ala. Acts, c. 6, §2 (1840).

2. Arizona—Howell Code, c. 10, §45 (1865).

3. Arkansas—Ark. Rev. Stat., c. 44, div. III, Art. II, §6 (1838).

4. California—Cal. Sess. Laws, c. 99, §45, p. 233 (1849–1850).

5. Colorado (Terr.)—Colo. Gen. Laws of Terr. of Colo., 1st Sess., §42, pp. 296–297 (1861).

6. Connecticut—Conn. Stat., Tit. 20, §§14, 16 (1821). By 1868, this statute had been replaced by another abortion law. Conn. Pub. Acts, c. 71, §§1, 2, p. 65 (1860).

7. Florida—Fla. Acts 1st Sess., c. 1637, subc. 3, §§10, 11, subc. 8, §§9, 10, 11 (1868), as amended, now Fla. Stat. Ann. §§782.09, 782.10, 797.01, 797.02, 782.16 (1965).

8. Georgia—Ga. Pen. Code, 4th Div., §20 (1833).

9. Kingdom of Hawaii—Hawaii Pen. Code, c. 12, §§1, 2, 3 (1850).

10. Idaho (Terr.)—Idaho (Terr.) Laws, Crimes and Punishments §§33, 34, 42, pp. 441, 443 (1863).

11. Illinois—Ill. Rev. Criminal Code §§40, 41, 46, pp. 130, 131 (1827). By 1868, this statute had been replaced by a subsequent enactment. Ill. Pub. Laws §§1, 2, 3, p. 89 (1867).

12. Indiana—Ind. Rev. Stat. §§1, 3, p. 224 (1838). By 1868 this statute had been superseded by a subsequent enactment. Ind. Laws, c. LXXXI, §2 (1859).

13. Iowa (Terr.)—Iowa (Terr.) Stat., 1st Legis., 1st Sess., §18, p. 145 (1838). By 1868, this statute had been superseded by a subsequent enactment. Iowa (Terr.) Rev. Stat., c. 49, §§10, 13 (1843).

14. Kansas (Terr.)—Kan. (Terr.) Stat., c. 48, §§9, 10, 39 (1855). By 1868, this statute had been superseded by a subsequent enactment. Kan. (Terr.) Laws, c. 28, §§9, 10, 37 (1859).

15. Louisiana—La. Rev. Stat., Crimes and Offenses §24, p. 138 (1856).

16. Maine—Me. Rev. Stat., c. 160, §§11, 12, 13, 14 (1840).

17. Maryland—Md. Laws, c. 179, §2, p. 315 (1868).

18. Massachusetts—Mass. Acts & Resolves, c. 27 (1845).

19. Michigan—Mich. Rev. Stat., c. 153, §§32, 33, 34, p. 662 (1846).

20. Minnesota (Terr.)—Minn. (Terr.) Rev. Stat., c. 100, §§10, 11, p. 493 (1851).

21. Mississippi—Miss. Code, c. 64, §§8, 9, p. 958 (1848).

22. Missouri—Mo. Rev. Stat., Art. II, §§9, 10, 36, pp. 168, 172 (1835).

23. Montana (Terr.)—Mont. (Terr.) Laws, Criminal Practice Acts §41, p. 184 (1864).

24. Nevada (Terr.)—Nev. (Terr.) Laws, c. 28, §42, p. 63 (1861).

25. New Hampshire—N. H. Laws, c. 743, §1, p. 708 (1848).

26. New Jersey—N. J. Laws, p. 266 (1849).

27. New York—N. Y. Rev. Stat., pt. 4, c. 1, Tit. 2, §§8, 9, pp. 12–13 (1828). By 1868, this statute had been superseded. N. Y. Laws, c. 260, §§1-6, pp. 285–286 (1845); N. Y. Laws, c. 22, §1, p. 19 (1846).

28. Ohio—Ohio Gen. Stat. §§111(1), 112(2), p. 252 (1841).

29. Oregon—Ore. Gen. Laws, Crim. Code, c. 43, §509, p. 528 (1845–1864).

30. Pennsylvania—Pa. Laws No. 374, §§87, 88, 89 (1860).

31. Texas—Tex. Gen. Stat. Dig., c. VII, Arts. 531–536, p. 524 (Oldham & White 1859).

32. Vermont—Vt. Acts No. 33, §1 (1846). By 1868, this statute had been amended. Vt. Acts No. 57, §§1, 3 (1867).

33. Virginia—Va. Acts, Tit. II, c. 3, §9, p. 96 (1848).

34. Washington (Terr.)—Wash. (Terr.) Stats., c. II, §§37, 38, p. 81 (1854).

35. West Virginia—See Va. Acts., Tit. II, c. 3, §9, p. 96 (1848); W. Va. Const., Art. XI, par. 8 (1863).

36. Wisconsin—Wis. Rev. Stat., c. 133, §§10, 11 (1849). By 1868, this statute had been superseded. Wis. Rev. Stat., c. 164, §§10, 11; c. 169, §§58, 59 (1858).

2. Abortion laws in effect in 1868 and still applicable as of August 1970:

  1.   Arizona (1865).

  2.   Connecticut (1860).

  3.   Florida (1868).

  4.   Idaho (1863).

  5.   Indiana (1838).

  6.   Iowa (1843).

  7.   Maine (1840).

  8.   Massachusetts (1845).

  9.   Michigan (1846).

  10.   Minnesota (1851).

  11.   Missouri (1835).

  12.   Montana (1864).

  13.   Nevada (1861).

  14.   New Hampshire (1848).

  15.   New Jersey (1849).

  16.   Ohio (1841).

  17.   Pennsylvania (1860).

  18.   Texas (1859).

  19.   Vermont (1867).

  20.   West Virginia (1863).

  21.   Wisconsin (1858).

Stem Cell Timeline

14th–13th century BC	Manava-Dharma-Sastra, sacred code of the Hindus, holds that the fetus results from the mixing of two seeds from the parents.
6th century BC	Greek physicians suggest studying the developing embryo within the chicken egg as a means of investigating embryology.
5th century BC	Anaxagoras of Clazomenae and Empedocles of Acragas, both of the Pythagorean School, assert that the developing offspring is the result of mixing two seeds from the parents.
5th century BC	Hippocrates believes that all parts of the body contain both the male and the female principles.
4th century BC	Aristotle promotes preformation and epigenesis; he believes that life begins 40 days after conception.
4th century BC	Herophilus of Alexandria claims that women have testes, and that the female genitalia are inverted versions of the male.
2nd century BC	Soranus determines that females are imperfect versions of males.
2nd century BC	Galen determines that the seeds of both man and woman contribute to the offspring.
1500s	Andreas Versalius echoes the idea that the woman's reproductive tract is an inverted version of the man's tract.
1561	Gabriele Fallopio describes the uterine tubes and egg follicles.
1619	Girolamo Fabrici investigates embryos and is considered the father of embryology.
1651	William Harvey studies embryology and casts doubt on Aristotle's theories of reproduction.
1672	Regnier de Graaf (1641–1673) is credited with naming the ovaries and finding the corpus luteum.

1600s	Bitter disputes arise between those who believe in preformation and those who believe in epigenesis.
1700	Anton van Leeuwenhoek (1632–1723), inventor of the microscope, views little animalcules (spermatic worms).
1712	Rene-Antoine Ferchault de Reaumur presents a paper on the regeneration of crayfish limbs to the French Academy.
1740–1744	Abraham Trembly finds that the hydra can regrow its severed heads.
1745	Charles Bonnet observes that the eyes of salamanders will regenerate, and also discovers the phenomenon called parthenogenesis.
1750	Lazarro Spallanzani investigates how salamanders are also able to regrow limbs, tails, and jaws.
1759	Casper Friedrich Wolff publishes an article titled "Theory of Generation," in which he argues that organs of the body do not exist in some preexistent form at the beginning of gestation but develop from some undifferentiated material through a series of steps.
1700s	A movement called natural philosophy adopts many of Wolff's ideas, leading to the development of cell theory during the nineteenth century.
1822	Etienne Geoffrey Saint-Hilaire publishes two volumes of the first detailed work on the study of malformations. His son Isadore invents the term *teratology*.
1827	Karl Ernst von Baer is the first to note a resemblance between dog and bird embryos as they develop.
1838	Mattias Schleiden and Theodor Schwann determine that the cell is the basic unit of life.
1855	Rudolph Virchow observes that every cell comes from other cells.
1875	Belgian zoologist Edouard Van Beneden (1845–1910) describes the early phases of embryonic development and finds what is now known as the blastocyst. He also describes the three basic layers of the blastocyst.
1890s	Wilhelm Roux introduces the concept of "developmental mechanics," which argues that embryologists must adopt experimental tools and the laws of chemistry and physics.
1890s	Hans Adolph Dreisch concludes that at some level all parts of the embryo are the same and that any given cell is a function of the whole.
1890	Walter Heape transfers a fertilized egg from a mother Angora rabbit to a foster mother rabbit of the Belgian line.

1899	Jacques Loeb establishes the first clear case of artificial parthenogenesis by pricking a frog's egg with a needle.
1912	Albert Brachet founds the famous Brussels School of embryology, which supports strongly the ideas of the new science of developmental mechanics.
1933	Thomas Hunt Morgan wins the Nobel Prize for his work in developmental genetics.
1930	Amniocentesis is first performed as a way to relate the condition of the developing embryo to the health of the baby.
1936	Gregory Pincus activates rabbit eggs by changing temperature and chemical exposure.
1953	Leroy Stevens goes to Jackson Laboratories and begins to research teratomas.
25 April 1953	James D. Watson and Francis H. Crick publish a one-page paper in the journal *Nature*, "The Molecular Structure of Nucleic Acids," in which they describe deoxyribonucleic acid (DNA).
1956	W. K. Whitten develops an eight-cell mouse embryo to the blastocyst stage.
1959	The first report of a rabbit produced from in vitro fertilization comes from the United States.
1961	Till and McCullough identify the hematopoietic cell that has the ability to renew itself and to differentiate into several cell types.
1964	Barry Pierce demonstrates that single undifferentiated cells isolated from one of the mouse teratomas and injected into normal mice can cause tumors that have the tissues of all three major germ layers.
1968	R. G. Edwards and B. D. Bavister fertilize the first human egg in a test tube.
1971	G. B. Pierce and Carol Wallace find similar differentiated and undifferentiated stem cells in squamous cell carcinoma, a type of skin cancer.
22 January 1973	The U.S. Supreme Court decides in *Roe v. Wade* to strike down the Texas law that made abortion a crime.
25 July 1978	R. G. Edwards and gynecologist P. Steptoe deliver the first test-tube baby, Louise Joy Brown.
May 1979	The Ethics Advisory Committee appointed by U.S. Congress concludes that research involving embryos is ethical, provided that the research does not take place after fourteen days of development and that all gamete donors are married couples.

1980	With the expiration of the Ethics Advisory Board charter, no channel exists to review proposals for federal funding for human embryo research, so during the 1980s no action is taken.
1980s	English investigators attempting to extract stem cells from human embryos find that stem cells can teach them about early development.
1981	Gail R. Martin and a team of scientists isolate embryonal carcinoma (EC) cells that have stable chromosomes and did not cause cancer.
1983	Ariff Bongso announces Asia's first test-tube baby and helps make IVF routine.
1987	Christopher Graham at Oxford studies the biological (genetic) factors in human embryos that regulate their potent cells, but has not considered therapeutic uses.
1988	Cord blood is used to cure Fanconi's anemia, a type of inherited blood disorder.
1989	Bongso produces the world's first micromanipulation baby.
1990s	Marshall Urist discovers bone morphogenetic protein (BMP) and revolutionizes orthopedics.
1991	President Bill Clinton takes office and encourages Congress to pass legislation that nullifies the requirement for EAB approval of federal funding for in vitro and embryo research.
1991	John Connolly injects a patient's own marrow and finds that the adult bone marrow cells assist in healing the patient's tibial fractures.
1992	Bongso leads a team that produces the world's first babies to be implanted as blastocysts, after the five-day development period.
1993	The Revitalization Act of 1993 (PL 103-43) allows NIH to propose funding in the area of stem cell research for the first time in 15 years.
1994	Bongso becomes the first to isolate stem cells from a five-day-old embryo and to document that these cells could transform themselves into any cell in the human body.
1996	Congress enacts the Dickey Amendment, named after Arkansas Rep. Jay Dickey, which prohibits federal funding for human embryo research.
1997	Ian Wilmut and his team at Roslin Institute in Edinburgh, Scotland clone the sheep named Dolly.

1998	James Thomson derives human embryonic stem cells (ESCs) from the inner cell mass and cultures them through many passages.
1998	John Gearhart produces embryonic stem cells from aborted fetuses.
2001	The Human Embryo Research Panel is formed with 19 members.
2001	Donald Orlic finds that injection of bone marrow into injured hearts promotes restoration of function.
9 August 2001	George W. Bush, in his first major public policy address, announces that federal funding will be available for the first time for research involving certain lines of embryo-derived stem cells.
2002	Bongso announces that his team has successfully grown a human embryonic stem cell (hESC) line entirely without mouse cells, and he founds Embryonic Stem Cell International (ECI) to distribute these cells.
April 2004	206 members of the House of Representatives sign a letter urging President Bush to modify his August 2001 executive order that limits federal research funds to preexisting stem cell lines.
November 2004	California citizens approve Proposition 71, a ten-year, $3 billion bond issue to fund stem cell research that includes embryonic stem cells.
20 December 2005	The Stem Cell Therapeutic and Research Act establishes cord blood stem cell banks to facilitate collection of human umbilical cord blood.
6 April 2006	Maryland Governor Robert L. Ehrlich signs legislation to authorize $15 million for both adult and embryonic stem cell research in the coming year.

Glossary

Abortion The premature termination of pregnancy before birth. A *spontaneous abortion* is the same thing as a miscarriage; an *induced abortion* is caused by a woman herself or by another person, usually a medical doctor.

Adult stem cells Undifferentiated cells found in differentiated adult tissue that can renew themselves and differentiate to yield all the specialized cell types of the tissue from which they originated

Allograft A graft transplanted from one individual to another, genetically different, member of the same species

Amniocentesis A procedure performed after the sixteenth week of pregnancy in which a needle is inserted to withdraw amniotic fluid for study for genetic or other birth defects

Astrocyte A star-shaped neuroglial cell

Autograft A graft obtained from an individual's own cells or body

Autologous Something that had its origin within the individual

Bioethics The study of norms of conduct that should govern research and clinical applications of biomedical knowledge

B lymphocytes Cells of the immune system that are nonphagocytic

Blastocyst The early embryo before it implants in the uterus. In humans it forms on the fourth or fifth day after fertilization and contains a cluster of cells called the inner cell mass.

Blastula The early stage of embryonic development when two kinds of cells develop: inner cell mass and trophoblast

Cardiomyocytes Cells of the heart muscle

CD+ 34 cells Cells that are part of the immune system

Cell fate Future possible course of differentiation that leads to a given cell type

Cell fusion The process whereby the cell membrane between two juxtaposed cells breaks down and re-forms to incorporate the cytoplasm and nuclei of both cells into a single viable cell

Cell theory Theory that cells are the building blocks of every tissue and organ in the body

Child Term used after a fetus is born. Pro-life position refers to the developing human individual, beginning shortly after conception.

Chimera A mixture of two or more types of animals; originally from a Greek mythological character that was partly lion, serpent, and goat

Chondrocytes Cartilage cells

Chorionic membrane The membrane that is the outmost tissue of the embryo

Chorionic villus sampling (CVS) A tool used to diagnose genetic defects in the fetus as early as the ninth week of pregnancy. A flexible catheter extracts some cells from the villi on the chorion, the outermost embryonic layer.

Conceptus A useful term meaning "that which has been conceived," coined by Daniel Callahan (1970). This neutral term refers to the developing human, and avoids the emotional terms used by different sides of the abortion issue.

Consequential In the argumentation of ethics, a term meaning the end result; same as teleological

Culture medium A material used for cell growth

Dedifferentiation The process in which adult cells become embryo cells

Deontology Duty-based reasons to perform an action, which may be based on religious command or which may stem from a sense of the rights of humans

Deoxyribonucleic acid (DNA) A long polymer that encodes for an organism's genes, formed by linking several kinds of nucleotides

Differentiation The process whereby an unspecialized early embryonic cell acquires the features of a specialized cell, such as a heart, liver, or muscle cell

Ectoderm The upper, outermost part of the three primitive germ layers of the embryo that will give rise to the skin, hair, nails, nerve, brain, and eye

Embryoid bodies Collections of hundreds of cells that resemble early embryos and that are produced by growing ES cells in the presence of retinoic acid. These bodies contain neural tube-like structures and have been successfully used to repair the damaged spinal cords of rats

Embryology The study of the development of offspring, from fertilization of the egg to birth

Embryo In humans, the developing individual from the second week through the end of the eighth week of gestation, when it becomes know as a fetus

Embryonal carcinoma cell (ECC) The stem cell that has developed into wildly growing cancerous cells

Embryonic germ stem cells (EGSCs) Cells found in the gonadal ridge of the embryo or fetus that normally develop into gametes—sperm and egg

Embryonic induction Starting the process of developing an embryo

Embryonic stem cells (ESCs) Primitive undifferentiated cells from the embryo that have the potential to become any of a wide variety of specialized cell types

Endoderm The lower, inner layer of the three primitive germ layers of the embryo that will give rise to the respiratory system, gastrointestinal tract, liver, pancreas, and bladder

Endothelial progenitor cells Cells that are precursors of the endothelium

Ensoulment Ethical or religious term used to describe when a being becomes human

Epigenesis The theory that the embryo develops in stages; opposed to the theory of preformation

Epithelial cells Skin cells

Erythrocytes Red blood cells

Ex vivo Latin term meaning "out of the body"

Fetus In humans, the developing embryo, from the eighth week until birth

Gamete A reproductive germ cell that unites to form a new offspring; can be sperm or egg

Gastrula The embryo during the phase of gastrulation, when tissues are beginning to be organized

Gastrulation The period of embryonic development when the body plan is laid down

Gene A unit of heredity that is a segment of DNA and is located at a specific site on a chromosome

Genome The organism's full complement of genes, or DNA

Gonadal ridge A site in the early fetus where the precursors to sperm and eggs are formed

Graft-versus-host disease (GVHD) The immunological reaction that occurs when a person receives an implant that is rejected

Growth factor A small protein that can stimulate cells to grow

Hemangioblast A progenitor of both endothelial and hematopoietic lines

Hematopoietic cell A type of cell found in bone marrow and other tissues that possesses the defining characteristics of self-renewal

Hippocampus An area in the brain

Hippocratic Oath An oath taken by new physicians in which they swear that they will do no harm

Human leukocyte antigen (HLA) typing Typing to match HLA factors before implant; HLA proteins on white blood cells cause rejection in nonmatched types

Implantation Process by which the mammalian blastocyst physically connects with the uterus of the mother

Induction Process that occurs when cells communicate, or signal, the body plan

Infarct An area of tissue that dies as a result of lack of blood supplied to that it

Inner cell mass (ICM) The cluster of cells inside the blastocyst that give rise to the embryo and ultimately the fetus; source of embryonic stem cells

Institutional review board (IRB) The board of an institution that approves research protocols, monitoring in particular the possible abuse of human subjects

In vitro Latin for "in glass"; can refer to a laboratory dish or test tube

In vitro fertilization (IVF) The fertilization of an egg outside the body, usually using a petri dish technique, which helps infertile couples trying to have children

In vivo Latin for "in life"; can refer to something in the living subject or in the natural environment

Ischemia A condition that occurs when the blood supply through an artery is deficient

Kant's practical imperative An ethical precept that holds that one should not harm one person for the good of another

Karyotype A photomicrograph of the nucleus of a single cell that shows a systematized array of metaphase chromosomes

Knockout technology The process of genetically engineering a species to not have a gene or series of genes that produce certain characteristics

Lin cell A type of enriched mesenchymal stem cell

Lymphocytes Cells of the lymphatic system

Meiosis Cell division for the formation of gametes—eggs and sperm

Messenger RNA (mRNA) An RNA transcribed from a gene that is used as the gene template to synthesize a protein

Mesenchymal stem cells (mSCs) Cells that, given exposure to different inductive mechanisms, have the capacity to form different mesenchymal tissues

Mesoderm The middle of the three primitive germ layers, which will give rise to most of the cardiovascular system, blood cells, bone marrow, skeleton, smooth and striated muscles, and parts of the reproductive and excretory systems

Mitosis The process of cell division

Monocyte A type of white blood cell

Morula A solid mass of cells resembling a blackberry that results from the cleavage of an ovum

Multipotent The characteristic of a stem cell that allows it to give rise to a limited range of cell types in the body

Myocytes Muscle cells

Natural killer cell (NKC) A type of white blood cell that, along with T cells, directs the immune response

Neural induction Refers to the early events that lead to the formation of neuroepithelial cells of the neural tube, where progenitor cells give rise to neurons and glial cells

Neural patterning Developmental process in which neural precursors are given a position that enables them to give rise to subtypes of neurons

Neural plate A thickened band of ectoderm along the dorsal surface of an embryo that develops into the nervous system

Neural stem cells Stem cells found in the brain that have the ability to make all the different cells of the nervous system, including neurons, astrocytes, and oligodendrocytes

Neuroepithelial cell (NEC) A special epithelial cell that forms the nerve endings in the sense organs

Neuron A nerve cell

Oligodendrocytes Cells of the neuroglia

Oncogene A mutant form of a normal cellular gene that can transform a cell into a cancerous cell

Ontological Having to do with the structure of a human being over the course of the individual's progress through life

Orthobiologics Biological solutions to orthopedic problems

Osteoblast Cell type that is responsible for bone formation

Osteoclast Cell type that is responsible for absorption and removal of unwanted bone

Osteocytes Bone cells

Otic Referring to the ear

Parthenogenesis The process of tricking a nonfertilized egg into duplication of DNA to produce an all-female–derived embryonic stem cell

Parthenotes Unfertilized eggs that are stimulated by chemical or electrical impulses and have grown to the blastocyst state

Phagocyte A cell that has the ability to digest and destroy invading material

Phosphorylate Combining a phosphate with an organic compound, which can act like a switch to turn on various processes

Placenta The spongy lining of the uterus from which the embryo receives nourishment

Plasticity The characteristic of being able to differentiate, or change, from one type to another.

Pluripotent cell A cell that can generate every cell type found in the embryo and adult, but not the cells that support the embryo

Preformation The theory that fully formed individuals are present in either egg or sperm

Proliferation Multiplication many times; great expansion

Protein A major constituent of cells and organisms, made by linking together amino acids

Quickening The moment when a woman is first able to feel the fetus move

Regenerative, or reparative, medicine A branch of medicine that applies cell-based therapies to healing

Reprogramming When an adult cell is transformed into an embryonic stem cell

Schwann cells Cells of ectodermal origin that constitute part of the nervous system

Self-renewal The ability of an entity to multiply or expand itself to the point that its cells are replenished

Somatic stem cell A stem cell from a body cell (same as an adult stem cell)

Stem cell A cell that has the ability to divide indefinitely in culture and give rise to specialized cells

Stemness The stem cell's potential to generate multiple mature cell types

Striatum An area in the midbrain that controls motor coordination

Stroma cells A mixed population of cells that generate bone, cartilage, and fibrous connective tissue

Syncytium A mass of cells that joins another mass of cells

T lymphocyte A type of white blood cell that directs the immune response

Teleological In the argumentation of ethics, a justification for action based on the ends or outcomes that one desires, which may support the greatest good for the greatest number

Telomerase An enzyme that forms at the ends of telomeres after each round of cell division to prevent shortening of chromosomes

Telomere The end of a chromsome

Teratogeny The process of developing anomalies or monsters in the embryos of animals

Teratoma A rare form of cancer that has a mass of both undifferentiated, or stem, cells and differentiated cells such as hair or baby teeth cells

Therapeutic cloning The deliberate creation of a human organism by nuclear transfer (cloning) technology in order to produce an embryo that can be used to create a stem cell line that will not provoke an immune response and rejection

Tissue engineering Regeneration of bone using stem cells, growth factors, and a scaffold (or matrix) to support the formation of bone

Totipotent cell The most versatile type of stem cell that can form other cells

Transcription The copying of a DNA sequence into RNA, catalyzed by a polymerase

Transcriptional factor A general term referring to a wide assortment of proteins needed to initiate or regulate transcription

Trophoblast A general term that describes all cell types of the developing and mature placenta, derived from the trophectoderm

Unipotent cells Those cells in the adult organism that are capable of developing along only one line

Utilitarian In the argumentation of ethics, a type of reasoning based on usefulness that justifies the end if it will produce a useful result

Ultrasonic testing A noninvasive sound (i.e., echo) test that is performed by at least twelve weeks after conception to acquire information.

Variolation Inoculation with smallpox by scratching into the skin the ooze of another smallpox patient's sores

Viability Occurs in a developing organism at some moment between the twenty-sixth and twenty-eighth week of gestation, at which time the conceptus is considered viable (i.e., able to survive outside the mother's womb). (Birth occurs between the thirty-ninth and fortieth week of pregnancy.)

Xenograft Graft of material from one body to another, sometimes associated with animal material

Zona pellucida Outer membrane of the blastocyst

Zygote A cell or group of cells that results from the union of sperm and egg cells; the fertilized egg

Further Reading

Alexandre, Henri. 2001. "A History of Mammalian Embryological Research." *International Journal of Developmental Biology* 45: 457–467.

Anderson, Arthur O. 2006. "A Brief History of Military Contribution to Ethical Standards for Research Involving Human Subjects." April 5, 2006. http://www.geocities.com/artnscience/jm4-primr.html.

Ariff Bongso. 2005. February 2, 2006. http://www.stemcell.edu.sg/ariff.htm.

Armon, Carmel. 2005. "Guest Editorial: January 2005 Stem Cell Research and Amytrophic Lateral Sclerosis." *Medscape Neurology and Neurosurgery* 7 (1). March 5, 2006. http://www.medscape.com/viewarticle/496732_print.

Ault, Alicia. 2004. "Tapping a Stem Cell Goldmine. *The Scientist* 18 (23): 38–39.

Baker, Robert. 1999. "Perspectives on the Professions." April 6, 2006. http://ethics.iit.edu/perspectives/pers19_1fall99_2.html.

BBC. 2005. "Applications Flood Stem Cell Ban." November 2, 2005. http://newsvote.bbc.co.uk/mpapps/pagetools/print/news.bbc.co.uk/2/hi/science/nature/4396.

Boggs, Will. 2005. "Stem Cells Aid Spinal Cord-Injured Mice." September 20, 2005. http://today.reuters.com/PrinterFriendlyPopup.aspx?type=healthNews&storyID=uri:2005.

Bourley, Jeffrey. 2005. "U. Cincinnati Researchers Discover Efficient Stem Cell Harvesting Technique." *Drug Discovery News* September: 21–22.

Broxmeyer, Hal E. 2006. "Cord Blood Hematopoietic Stem and Progenitor Cells." In *Essentials of Stem Cell Biology* (pp. 133–137), ed. Robert Lanza. Burlington, MA: Elsevier Academic Press.

Bush, George. "Remarks by the President on Stem Cell Research." White House Press Office, August 9, 2001. http://www.whitehouse.gov/news/releases/2001/08/200108092.html.

Callahan, Daniel. 1970. *Abortion, Law, Choice, and Morality*. New York: Macmillan.

Cameron, David. Fall 2004. "Life, Death, and Stem Cells." *Paradigm.* Cambridge, MA:Whitehead Institute for Biomedical Research.

Cancelas, Jose, and David Williams. 2005. "New Finding May Aid Adult Stem Cell Collection." http://healthnews.uc.edu/publications/findings/?/1653/1661/.

Cepko, Connic, and Danna M. Fekete. 2006. "Semspru Epithelium of the Eye and Ear." In *Essentials of Stem Cell Biology* (pp. 161–168), ed. Robert Lanza. Burlington, MA: Elsevier Academic Press.

"Childbirth by Choice Trust." April 15, 2006. http://www.cbtrust.com/history_law_religion.php.

"Chondrogen Clinical Trial Information." March 5, 2006. http:www.osiristx.com/clinical_trials_chondrogen.php.

Clement, A. M., et al. 2003. "Wild Type Neuronal Cells Extend Survuval of SOD1 Neurons in ALS Mice." *Science* 302 (5642), 113–117. http://www.sciencemag.org/cgi/content/abstract/302/5642/113.

"The Color of Life." 2005. *Research at Children's Hospital & Research Center at Oakland.* Press kit: www.childrenshospitaloakland.org.

Colson, Charles. 2006. "Following the Money: Embryonic Stem Cells and Big Buck." In *Florida Baptist Witness.* April 6. Jacksonville, FL: Florida Baptist Convention, 10.

Committee on the Biological and Biomedical Applications of Stem Cell Research. 2002. *Stem Cells and the Future of Regenerative Medicine.* Washington, D.C.: National Academy Press.

Cook, Gareth, and Carey Goldberg. 2005. "Newly Created Cells Wouldn't Harm Embryo" (reprint from the *Boston Globe*). *The Orange County Register* August 23: 6.

"Cooper and Coriell Pioneer Stem Cell Heart Research; Partnership Changes the Face of Research for Cardiac Care." March 6, 2006. http://media.prnewswire.com/en/jsp/includes/contents/printable.jsp?resourceid=3153913.

Cooper, Melinda. 2004. Regenerative Medicine: Stem Cells and the Science of Monstrosity. *BMJ Publishing Group Ltd and Institute of Medical Ethics* 30:12–22. http://mh.bmjjournals.com/cgi/content/abstract/30/1/12. accessed March 6, 2006.

Cyranoski, David, and Declan Butler. 2006. "Stem Cells Found in Mouse Testes." March 27, 2006. news@natture.com http://www.nature.com/news/2006/060320/pf/060430-10_pf.html.

DiCoppi, Paolo, et al. 2006. "Amniotic Fluid-Derived Pluripotential Cells." In *Essentials of Stem Cell Biology* (pp. 127–131), ed. Robert Lanza. Burlington, MA: Elsevier Academic Press.

Dolinski, Catherine. 2005. "Cross-Country Wheelchair Trip To Raise Stem Cell Funds. *Ocala Star Banner* September 5: 1B and 3B.

Dreifus, Claudia. 2006. "At Harvard's Stem Cell Center, the Barriers Run Deep and Wide." January 24, 2006. http://www.nytimes.com/2006/01/24/science/24conv.html?_r=1&th=&emc=th&pagewant.

Dunstan, G. R. 1984. "Moral Status of the Human Embryo: A Tradition Recalled. *Journal of Medical Ethics* March 10(1): 38–44.

"Embryology: The History of Developmental and Generational Theory." 2002. In *World of Genetics*, Vol. I (pp. 226–227), ed. Lee and Brenda Lerner. Farmington Hills, MI: Gale Group.

Farley, Margaret A. 2006. "Stem Cell Research: Religious Considerations." In *Essentials of Stem Cell Biology* (pp. 495–501), ed. Robert Lanza. Burlington, MA: Elsevier Academic Press.

Green, Ronald. 2006. "Ethical Considerations." In *Essentials of Stem Cell Biology* (pp. 489–493), ed. Robert Lanza. Burlington, MA: Elsevier Academic Press.

Green, Ronald M. 2001. *The Human Embryo Research Debates*. New York: Oxford Press.

Hamilton, Pauline. 2003. "Autoimmune Stem Cells." *Drug & Market Development* 14 (1): 8–12.

"History of Regeneration Research." January 16, 2006. http://odelberglab.genetics. utah.edu/index.htm.

Hoffman, Joseph. 2001. "The Philosophy of Greek Medicine." In *Science and Its Times,* ed. Neil Schlager. Detroit, MI: Gale Group.

Hogan, Brigid. 2002. From talks at Vanderbilt University, "The Ethics of Human Stem Cell Research." Cited in Zoloth, Laurie. 2006. "The Ethics of Human Stem Cell Research: Immoral Cells, Moral Selves." In *Essentials of Stem Cell Biology* (pp. 479–488), ed. Robert Lanza. Burlington, MA: Elsevier Academic Press.

Huang, Jerry, et al. 2006. "Orthopedic Applications of Stem Cells." In *Essentials of Stem Cell Biology* (pp. 449–456), ed. Robert Lanza. Burlington, MA: Elsevier Academic Press.

Hyun, Insoo. 2006. "Magic Eggs and the Frontier of Stem Cell Science." *Hastings Center Report* 36(2): 6–19.

Jonsen, Albert. 2000. *A Short History of Medical Ethics*. New York: University Press.

Klatzko, Arlene-Judith. 2000. "Embryo Stem Cells: Raw Material for Tissue Engineering." June 28, 2005. http://www.medscape.com/viewarticle/408763_print.

Klimanskaya, Irina, and Jill McMahon. 2006. "Approaches for Derivation and Maintenance of Human ES Cells: Detailed Procedures and Alternatives." In *Essentials of Stem Cell Biology* (pp. 287–298), ed. Robert Lanza. Burlington, MA: Elsevier Academic Press.

"Lab Grows Bladder From Cells of Patients." April 4, 2006. http://www.nytimes. com/aponline/us/AP-Regrown_Bladders.html.

Lanza, Robert, ed. 2006. *Essentials of Stem Cell Biology*. Burlington, MA: Elsevier Academic Press.

Lanza, Robert, ed. 2004. *Handbook of Stem Cells,* Vol. 1. Burlington, MA: Elsevier.

Lee, M. S., and Lill M. Makkar. 2004. "Stem Cell Transplantation in Myocardial Infarction." *Review of Cardiovascular Medicine* 5: 82–98.

Leor, J., et al. In press. "Human Umbilical Cord Blood-derivedCD 133+ Stem/Progenitor Cells for Myocardial Tissue Repair." *Circulation*. http://www.medscape.com/viewarticle/496380_print. Accessed March 5, 2006.

"Lernean Hydra." January 20, 2006. http://www.perseus.tufts.edu/Herakles/hydra.html.

Lewis, Ricki. 2005. "Stem Cells: An Emerging Portrait." *The Scientist* 19 (13): 14.

Lynch, Richard. 2002. "Milestones in Investigative Pathology" (excerpt). *American Society for Investigative Pathology* 5 (1).

Ma, D. R., et al. 2004. *Annals of Academic Medicine Singapore* 33 (6): 784–788.

Magner, Lois. 2000. "Developments in Embryology." In *Science and Its Times*, ed. Neil Schlager. Farmington Hills, MI: Gale Group.

Mariani, Sara. 2004. "Shaping the Fate of Stem Cells." *Medscape Molecular Medicine* 6(1). http://www.medscape.com/viewpublication/221. Accessed Jan. 10, 2006.

Moore, Mary Tyler, with S. Robert Levine. 2006. "It's Not About Curiosity, It's About Cures—Stem Cell Research: People Help Drive Progress" In *Essentials of Stem Cell Biology* (pp. 513–518), ed. Robert Lanza. Burlington, MA: Elsevier Academic Press.

"Morgan, Thomas Hunt." 2002. In *World of Genetics*, Vol. II (pp. 486–487), ed. Lee and Brenda Lerner. Farmington Hills, MI: Gale Group.

Murray, Thomas H. 2005. "In Brief: Will New Ways of Creating Stem Cells Dodge the Objection?" *Hastings Center Report* 35 (1): 8–9.

National Academies. 2005. *Guidelines for Human Embryonic Stem Cell Research.* Washington, D.C.: The National Academies Press.

National Institutes of Health. 2005. "Stem Cell Basics." June 28, 2005. http://stemcells.nih.gov/info/basics/basics2.asp.

Navigant Consulting. 2005. June 28, 2005. http://navigantconsulting.com.

News from the American Medical Association. 2006. "Preliminary Research Shows Promise for Using Stem Cell Transplantation to Treat Patients with Severe Lupus." April 6, 2006. http://www.medem.com/medlb/article_detailb_for_printer.cfm?article_ID=ZZZ3PBT39JE.

Niesen, Jim. 2006. Personal interview. March 10.

Odelberg Laboratory. 2005. "Research Interests." January 16, 2006. http://odelberglab.genetics.utah.edu/index.htm.

Ogawa, K., et al. 2004. "Transient Improvement of Left Ventricular Function After Peripheral Blood Stem Cell Transplantation in a Patient with Myelodysplastic Syndrome and Dilated Cardiomyopathy." *Circulation* 68: 958–960.

Orlic, D., et al. (2001). *Nature* 410: 701–705.

Panno, Joseph. 2005. *Stem Cell Research.* New York: Facts on File, Inc.

Pobojewski, Sally. 2005. "In Support of Medical Research with Human Embryonic Stem Cells. *Medicine at Michigan* Spring/Summer: 44–47.

"The Quest for Innovative Science." 2002. February 2, 2006. http://sciencecareers. sciencemag.org/layout/set/print/career_development/previous_issues/ar.

Reeve, Christopher. 2006. "Patient Advocacy." In *Essentials of Stem Cell Biology* (pp. 519–520), ed. Robert Lanza. Burlington, MA: Elsevier Academic Press.

Reinberg, Steven. 2005. "Banking on Stem Cells." *The Scientist* 19 (14): 22.

Ribbink, Kim. 2005. "Ideology vs. Science: The Stem Cell Battle." *PharmaVOICE* June: 42–50.

Saywell, Trish. 2002. "Stem Cell Secrets Unlocked." February 2, 2006. http:// www.feer.com/articles/2002/0210_24/free/p038innov.html.

Seoul National University Investigation Committee. 2006. *Final Report on Professor Woo Suk Huang's Research Allegations*, January 10, 2006. http://www. iht.com/articles/2006/01/10/asia/web.0110clone.text.php.

Singer, Emily. 2005. "Therapies Come Closer with Cleaner Stem Cell Lines." *Nature Medicine* 11 (4): 357.

Smith, A. G. 2001. "Embryo-Derived Stem Cells: Of Mice and Men." *Annual Review of Cell Developmental Biology* 17, 435–462.

Studer, Lorenz. 2006. "The Nervous System." In *Essentials of Stem Cell Biology* (pp. 149–156), ed. Robert Lanza. Burlington, MA: Elsevier Academic Press.

Thiroux, Jacques P. 2004. *Ethics Theory and Practice*. Upper Saddle River, NJ: Pearson/Prentice Hall.

Thomson, James, et al.1998 "Embryonic Stem Cell Lines Derived from Human Blastocysts." *Science* 282: 1145–1147.

"Time line of a Controversy: A Chronology of Woo Suk Hwang's Stem Cell Research." January 16, 2006. http://www.nature.com/news/2005/051219/pf/ 051219-3_pf.html.

Upjohn, Edward, et al. 2006. "Burns and Skin Ulcers." In Lanza, Robert, ed. *Essentials of Stem Cell Biology* (pp. 419–423), ed. Robert Lanza. Burlington, MA: Elsevier Academic Press.

Verfallie, Catherine. 2006 "Adult Stem Cells: Tissue Specific or Not?" In *Essentials of Stem Cell Biology* (pp. 23–28), ed. Robert Lanza. Burlington, MA: Elsevier Academic Press.

Wade, Nicholas. 2006. "Regrow Your Own." April 11, 2006. http://www.nytimes. com/2006/04/11/health/11regen.html?_r=2&oref=slogin&pagewanted.

Wade, Nicolas. 2005. "Ethicists Offer Advise for Testing Human Brain Cells in Primate. *New York Times* July 15: A12.

Whitehead Institute for Biomedical Research. 2005. "Rudolf Jaenisch, MD." February 2, 2006. http://www.wi.mit.edu/research/faculty/jaenisch.html.

Wininger, J. David. 2004. "Parthenogenetic Stem Cells." In *Essentials of Stem Cell Biology* (pp. 513–518), ed. Robert Lanza. Burlington, MA: Elsevier Academic Press.

Wold, Loren, et al. 2004. "Stem Cell Therapy for the Heart." March 5, 2006. http://www.medscape.com/viewarticle/496380_print.

The Yomiuri Shimbun. 2005. "Bone-Cell Therapy Let's Man Shed Artificial Heart" (reprint). *Orange County Register (California)* August 28: 27.

Young, Holly, Chunhui Xu, and Melissa Carpenter. 2006. "Feeder-Free Culture."
    In *Essentials of Stem Cell Biology* (pp. 317–323), ed. Robert Lanza. Burlington,
    MA: Elsevier Academic Press.
Zoloth, Laurie. 2006. "The Ethics of Human Stem Cell Research: Immoral Cells,
    Moral Selves." In *Essentials of Stem Cell Biology* (pp. 479–488), ed. Robert
    Lanza. Burlington, MA: Elsevier Academic Press.

INDEX

ABOUT THE AUTHOR

EVELYN B. KELLY, Ph.D., is a writer, educator, and community activist living in Ocala, Florida. She specializes in writing about the diseases and disorders of the nervous and endocrine systems and enjoys tackling cutting edge research. Throughout her years as a writer, she has written 10 books and over 400 articles, including *The Skeletal System* (2004) and *Obesity* (2006) for Greenwood Press. She is an adjunct professor of education at Saint Leo University in Florida and an international speaker on educational topics.